Easy Mediterranean Cookbook

Everyday Pasta Recipes for Healthy Living

Ben Cooper

Table of Contents

Rice Jambalaya

Preparation Time: 5 minutes
Cooking Time: 30 minutes
Servings: 8

Ingredients:

1 cup tomatoes, chopped
1 cup bell pepper, chopped
¼ cup carrot, chopped
1 tsp. cayenne pepper
4 cups chicken stock
1 cup of basmati rice
2 tbsp. olive oil
½ cup chickpeas, cooked

Directions:

1.Melt the olive oil and add carrot, bell pepper, and tomatoes.

2.Cook the vegetables for 10 minutes on medium heat.

3.Then add chicken stock, chickpeas, and rice.

4.Add cayenne pepper and stir the meal.

5.Close the lid and cook it for 20 minutes on low heat.

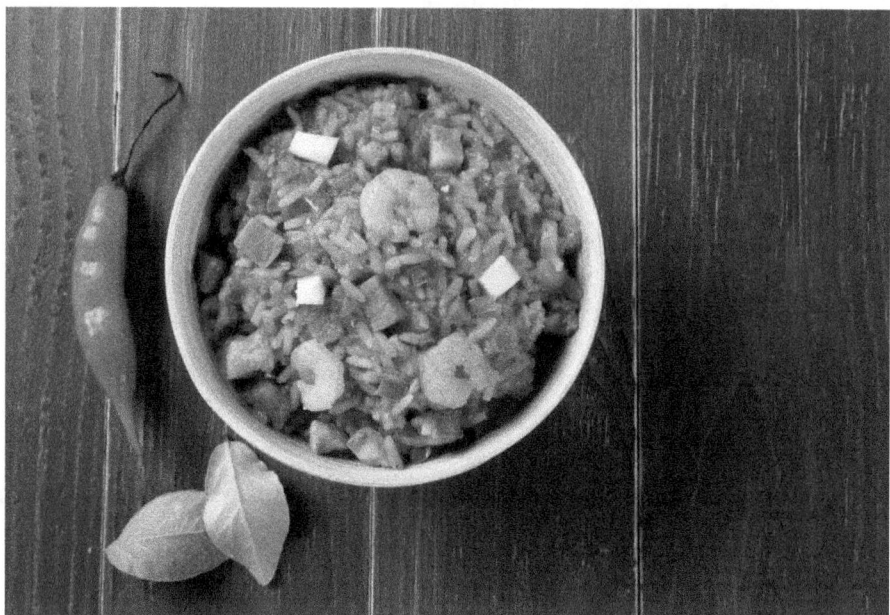

Jasmine Rice with Scallions

Preparation Time: 10 minutes
Cooking Time: 10 minutes
Servings: 6

Ingredients:

3 tbsp. olive oil
1 cup jasmine rice
2 tbsp. scallions, chopped
½ tsp. ground black pepper
2 tsp. lemon juice

Directions:

1.Cook the rice according to the directions of the manufacturer.

2.Then add scallions, olive oil, ground black pepper, and lemon juice.

3.Carefully stir the meal.

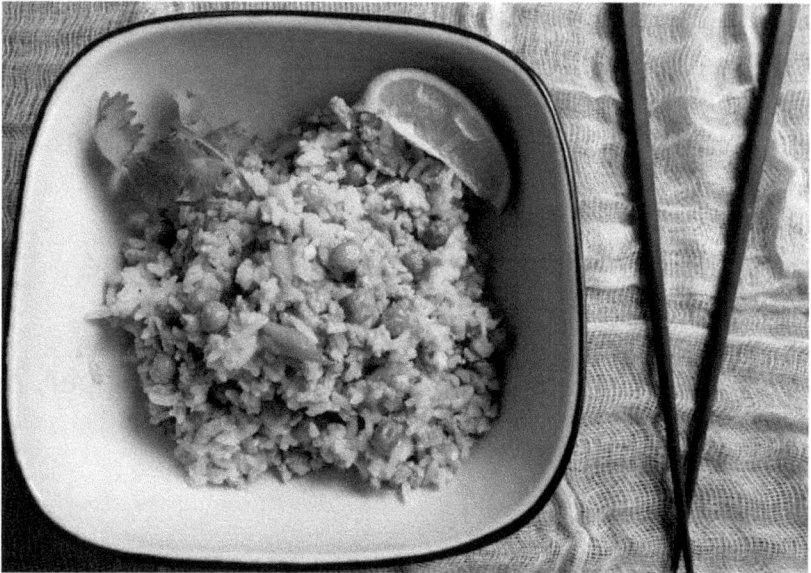

Cremini Mushrooms Pilaf

Preparation Time: 10 minutes
Cooking Time: 25 minutes
Servings: 6

Ingredients:

2 cups of water
½ cup white onion, diced
1 cup cremini mushrooms, chopped
1 cup of basmati rice
¼ tsp. lime zest, grated
2 oz goat cheese, crumbled
2 tbsp. olive oil

Directions:

1.Put rice in the saucepan.

2.Add water and cook for 15 minutes over the low heat.

3.Then roast the mushrooms with olive oil, lime zest, and white onion in the skillet until they are light brown.

4.Add the cooked mushrooms in the cooked rice. Stir well.

5.Top the meal with crumbled goat cheese.

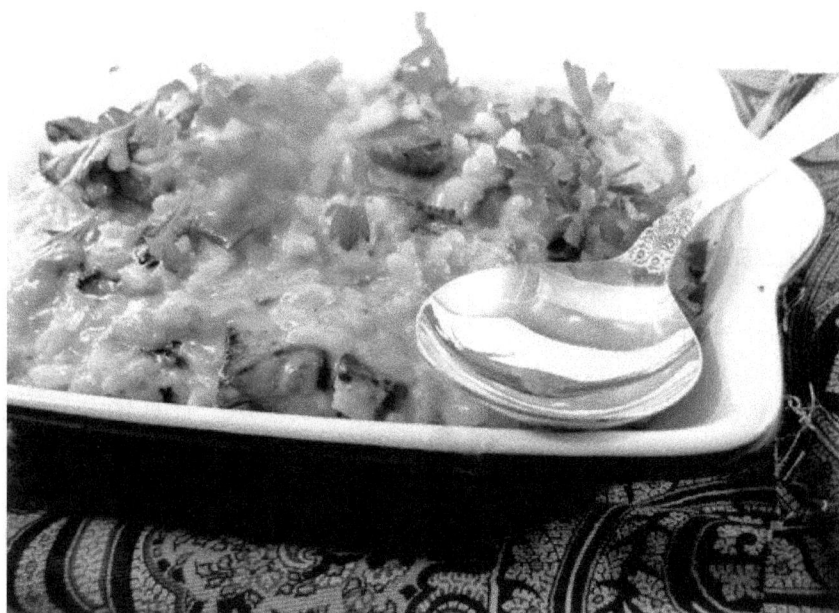

Vegetable Rice
Preparation Time: 10 minutes
Cooking Time: 30 minutes
Servings: 6

Ingredients:
2 cups wild rice
1 tsp. Italian seasonings
1 tbsp. olive oil
¼ cup carrot, diced
½ cup snap peas, frozen
5 cups of water

Directions:

1.Mix 4 cups of water and wild rice in the saucepan.

2.Cook the rice for 15 minutes or until the rice soaks all liquid.

3.Then heat the olive oil in the separated saucepan.

4.Add carrot and roast it until light brown.

5.Add snap peas, water, and rice.

6.Stir well and close the lid.

7.Cook the rice for 10 minutes.

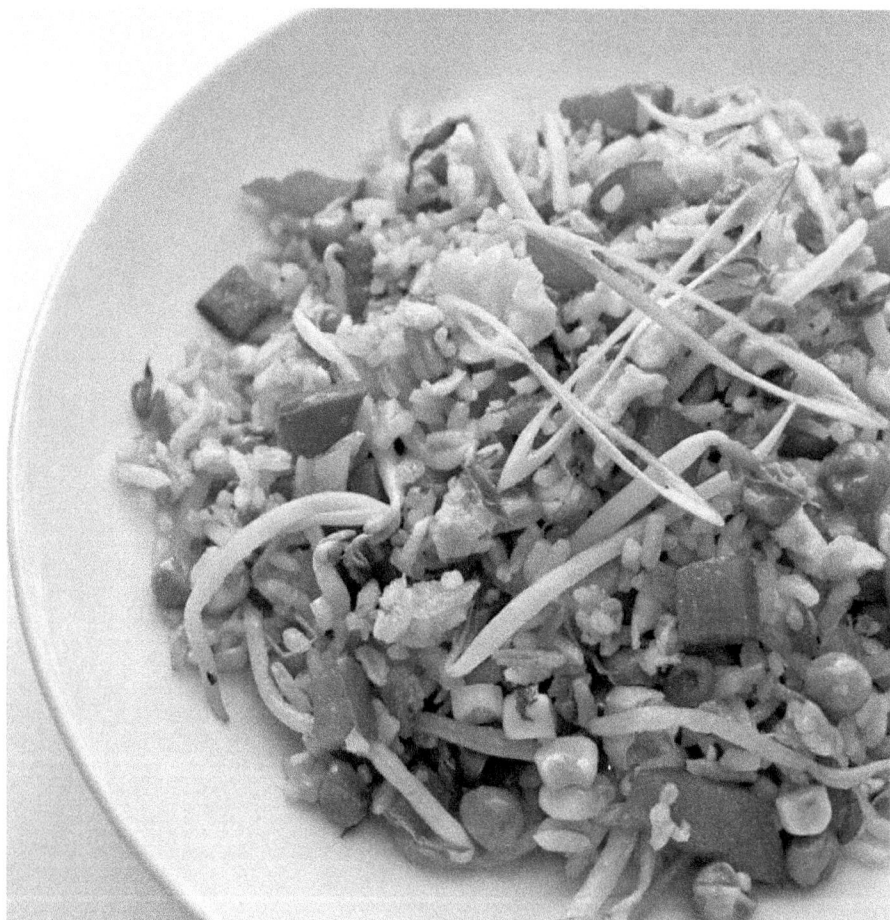

Tomato Rice

Preparation Time: 10 minutes
Cooking Time: 20 minutes
Servings: 4

Ingredients:

1 cup basmati rice
3 cups chicken stock
1 tsp. ground coriander
¼ tsp. dried thyme
2 tbsp. olive oil
2 tbsp. tomato paste

Directions:

1.Roast the rice with olive oil in the saucepan for 5 minutes. Stir it.

2.Then add thyme, coriander, and tomato paste.

3.Add water, mix the rice mixture, and close the lid.

4.Cook the rice for 15 minutes over the medium heat.

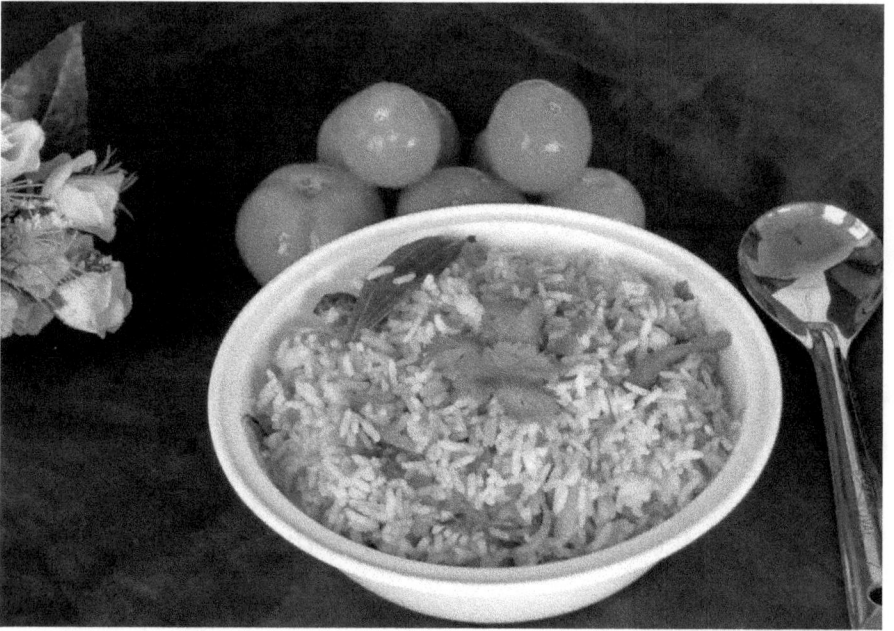

Rice with Grilled Tomatoes

Preparation Time: 10 minutes
Cooking Time: 20 minutes
Servings: 6

Ingredients:

1 cup of basmati rice cups chicken stock
1 tsp. olive oil
2 tomatoes, roughly sliced

Directions:

1.Sprinkle the tomatoes with olive oil and grill in the preheated to 400F grill for 1 minute per side.

2.Then cook rice with chicken stock for 15 minutes.

3.Transfer the cooked rice in the bowls and top with grilled tomatoes.

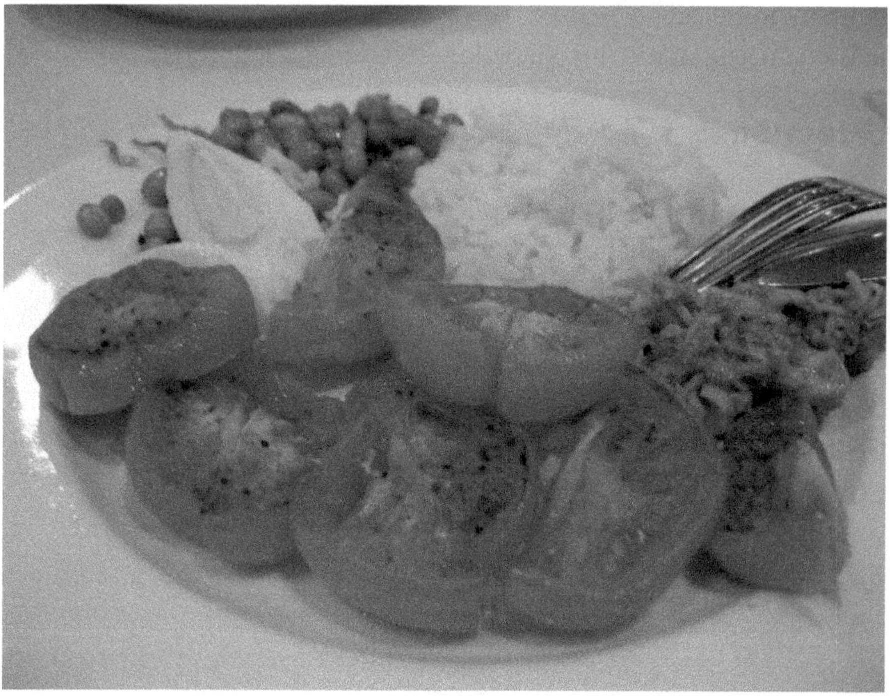

Rice and Meat Salad

Preparation Time: 10 minutes
Cooking Time: 0 minutes
Servings: 6

Ingredients:

1 cup white cabbage, shredded
1 cup long grain rice, cooked
8 oz beef steak, cooked, cut into the strips
1/3 cup plain yogurt
1 tsp. salt
1 tsp. chives, chopped

Directions:

1.Put cabbage and rice in the big bowl.

2.Add white rice and meat strips.

3.Then add plain yogurt, chives, and salt.

4.Stir the salad until homogenous.

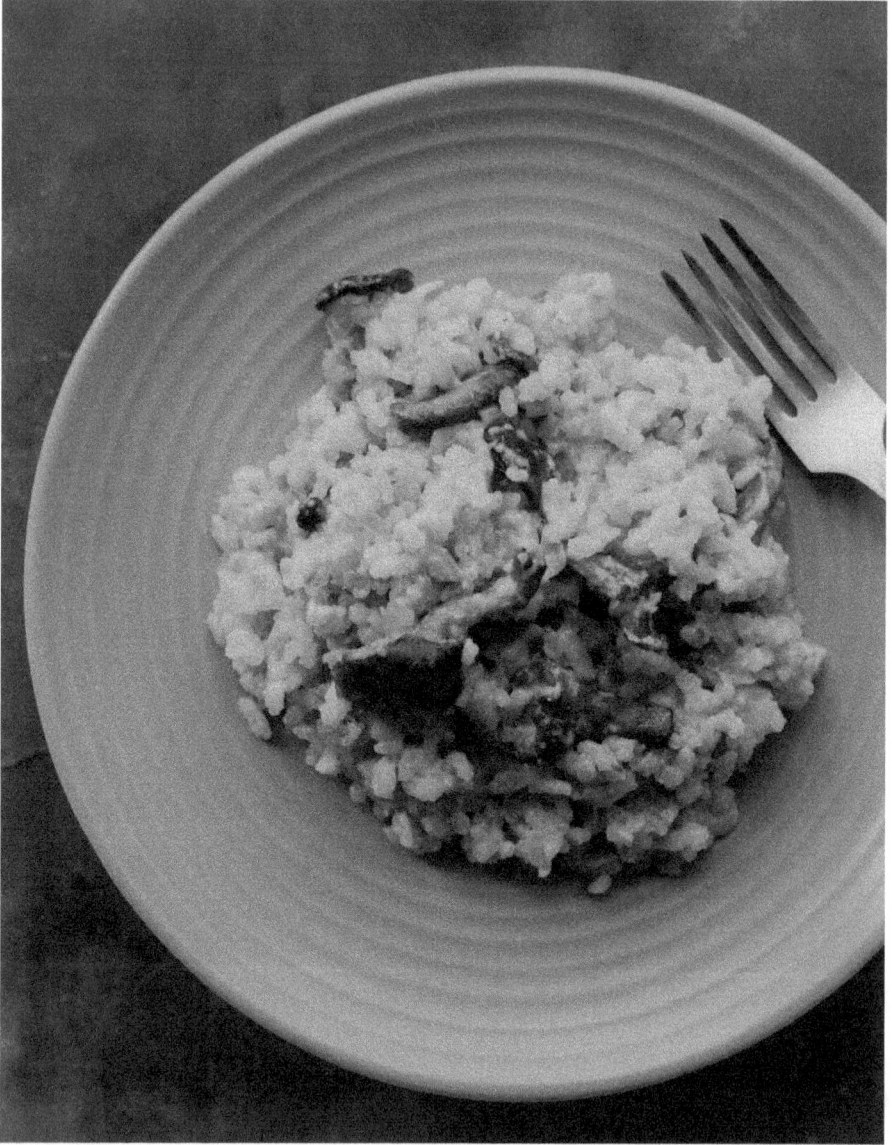

Rice Bowl

Preparation Time: 10 minutes
Cooking Time: 0 minutes
Servings: 6

Ingredients:

1 cup of basmati rice, cooked
4 oz beef sirloin, grilled
½ cup tomatoes, chopped
2 tbsp. soy sauce
1 tsp. ground paprika
2 oz scallions, sliced

Directions:

1.Put the cooked rice in the serving bowls.

2.Add beef sirloin, tomatoes, and scallions.

3.Then sprinkle the meal with soy sauce and ground paprika.

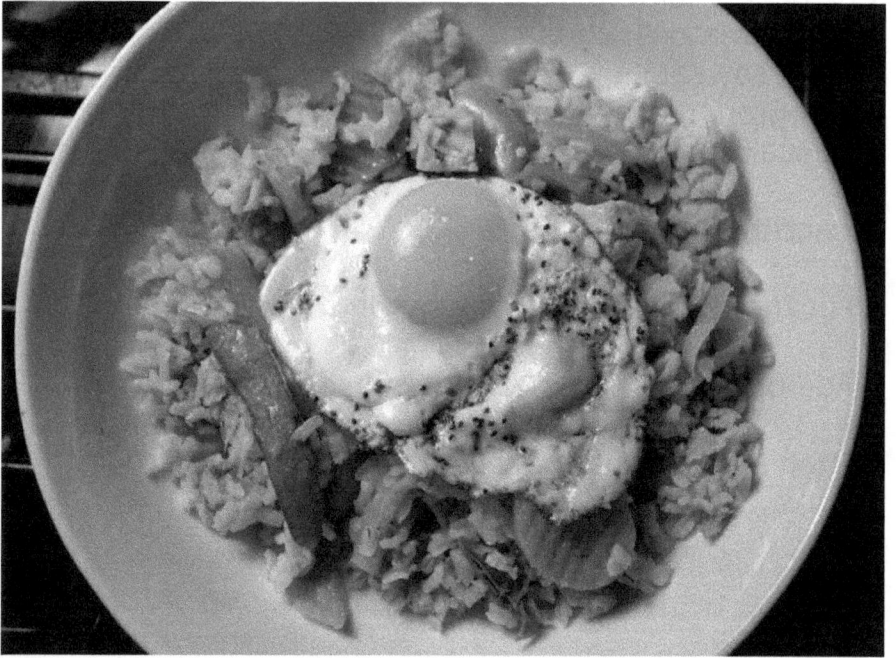

Zucchini Rice
Preparation Time: 10 minutes
Cooking Time: 25 minutes
Servings: 2

Ingredients:

½ cup of long grain rice
1 cup chicken stock
1 zucchini, cubed
1 tbsp. olive oil
1 tsp. curry powder
1 tbsp. raisins

Directions:

1.Mix rice and chicken stock in the saucepan and cook for 15 minutes or until the rice soaks the liquid.

2.Then heat the olive oil.

3.Add zucchini in the oil and roast for 5 minutes.

4.After this, sprinkle the zucchini with curry powder, add raisins and rice.

5.Carefully mix the rice and cook for 5 minutes.

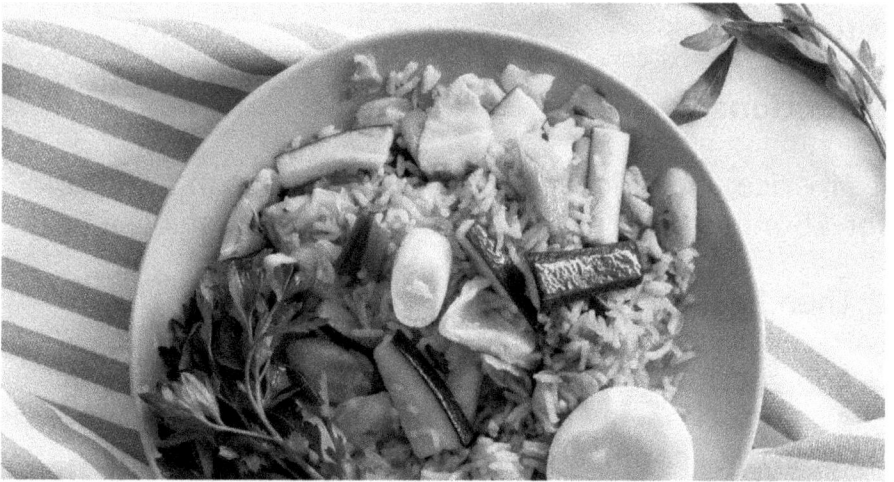

Rice Soup

Preparation Time: 10 minutes
Cooking Time: 20 minutes
Servings: 4

Ingredients:

3 cups chicken stock
½ lb. chicken breast, shredded
1 tbsp. chives, chopped
1 egg, whisked
½ white onion, diced
1 bell pepper, chopped
1 tbsp. olive oil
¼ cup arborio rice
½ tsp. salt
1 tbsp. fresh cilantro, chopped

Directions:

1.Pour olive oil in the stock pan and preheat it.

2.Add onion and bell pepper. Roast the vegetables for 3-4 minutes. Stir them from time to time.

3.After this, add rice and stir well.

4.Cook the ingredients for 3 minutes over the medium heat.

5.Then add chicken stock and stir the soup well.

6.Add salt and bring the soup to boil.

7.Add shredded chicken breast, cilantro, and chives. Add egg and stir it carefully.

8.Close the lid and simmer the soup for 5 minutes over the medium heat.

9.Remove the cooked soup from the heat.

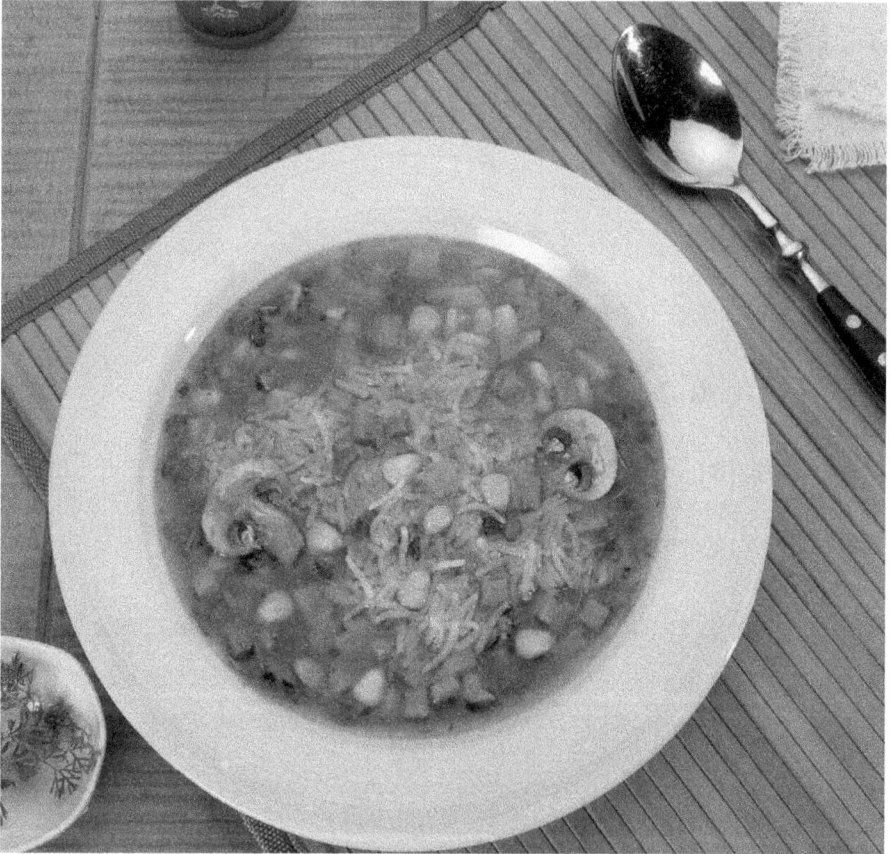

Rice with Prunes

Preparation Time: 5 minutes
Cooking Time: 20 minutes
Servings: 7

Ingredients:

1.5 cup basmati rice
3 tbsp. organic canola oil
5 prunes, chopped
¼ cup cream cheese
3.5 cups water
½ tsp. salt

Directions:

1.Mix water and basmati rice in the saucepan and boil for 15 minutes on low heat.

2.Then add cream cheese, salt, and prunes.

3.Stir the rice carefully and bring it to boil.

4.Add organic canola oil and cook for 1 minute more.

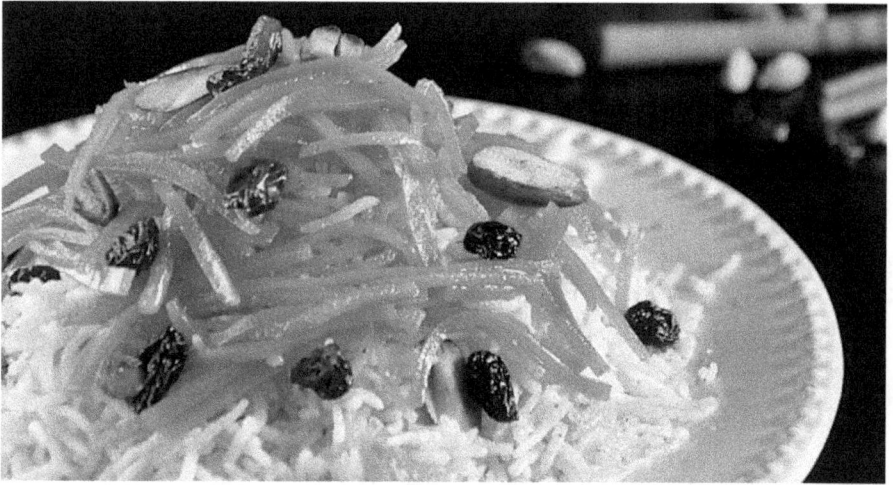

Rice and Fish Cakes

Preparation Time: 10 minutes
Cooking Time: 10 minutes
Servings: 6

Ingredients:

6 oz salmon, canned, shredded
1 egg, beaten
¼ cup of basmati rice, cooked
1 tsp. dried cilantro
½ tsp. chili flakes
1 tbsp. organic canola oil

Directions:

1.Mix salmon with egg, basmati rice, dried cilantro, and chili flakes.

2.Heat the organic canola oil in the skillet.

3.Make the small cakes from the salmon mixture and put in the hot oil.

4. Roast the cakes for 2 minutes per side or until they are light brown.

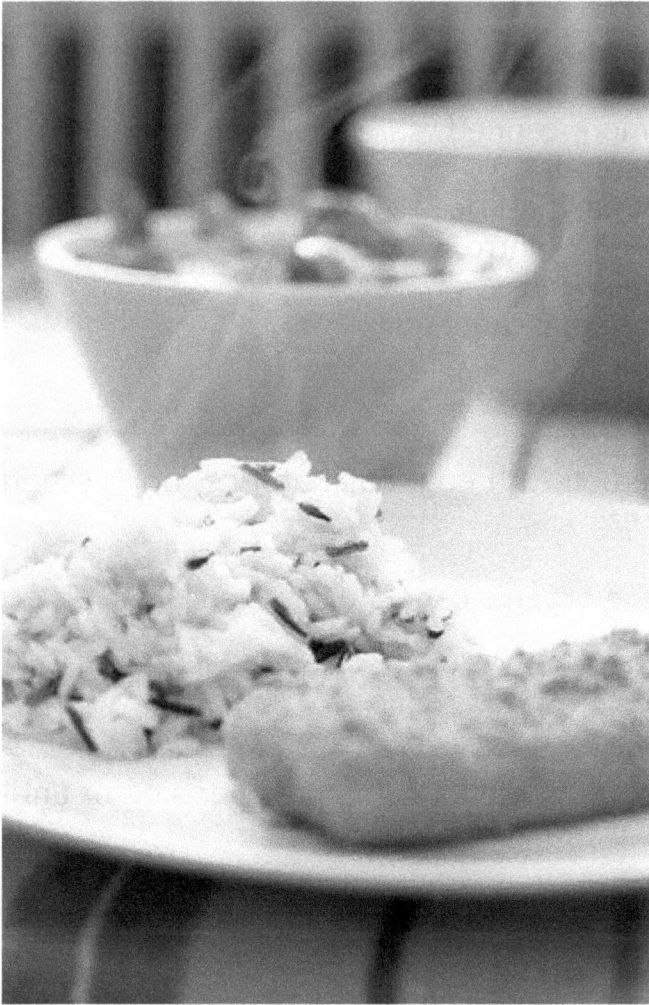

Salsa Rice

Preparation Time: 10 minutes
Cooking Time: 15 minutes
Servings: 6

Ingredients:

9 oz long grain rice
4 cups chicken stock
1 cup of salsa
2 tbsp. avocado oil

Directions:

1.Mix chicken stock and rice in the saucepan.

2.Cook the rice for 15 minutes on medium heat.

3.Then cool it to the room temperature and mix with avocado oil and salsa.

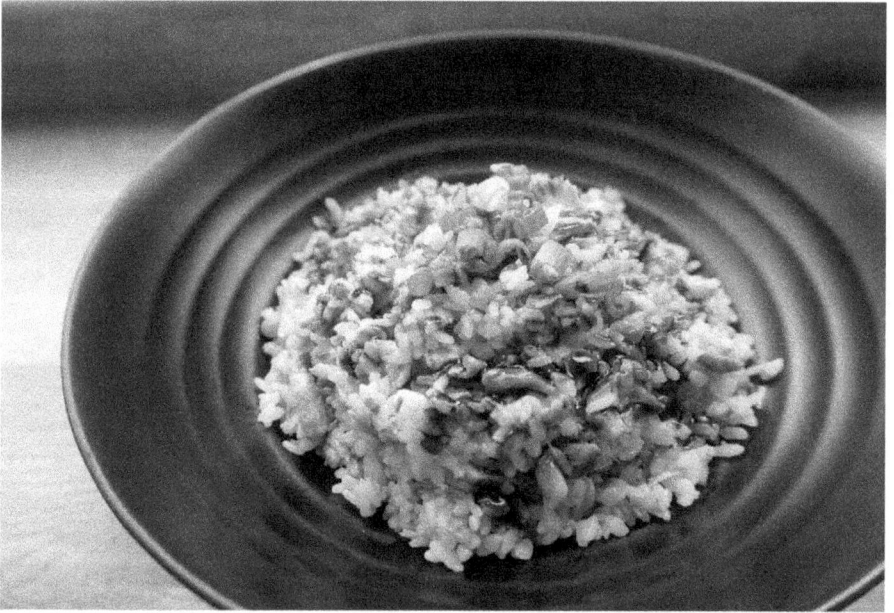

Seafood Rice

Preparation Time: 10 minutes
Cooking Time: 30 minutes
Servings: 4

Ingredients:

½ cup seafood mix, frozen
½ cup of long grain rice
3 cups of water
1 tbsp. olive oil
½ tsp. ground coriander

Directions:

1.Boil the rice with water for 15-18 minutes or until it soaks all water.

2.Then heat olive oil in the saucepan.

3.Add seafood mix and ground coriander. Cook the ingredients for 10 minutes on low heat.

4.Then add rice, stir well, and cook for 5 minutes more.

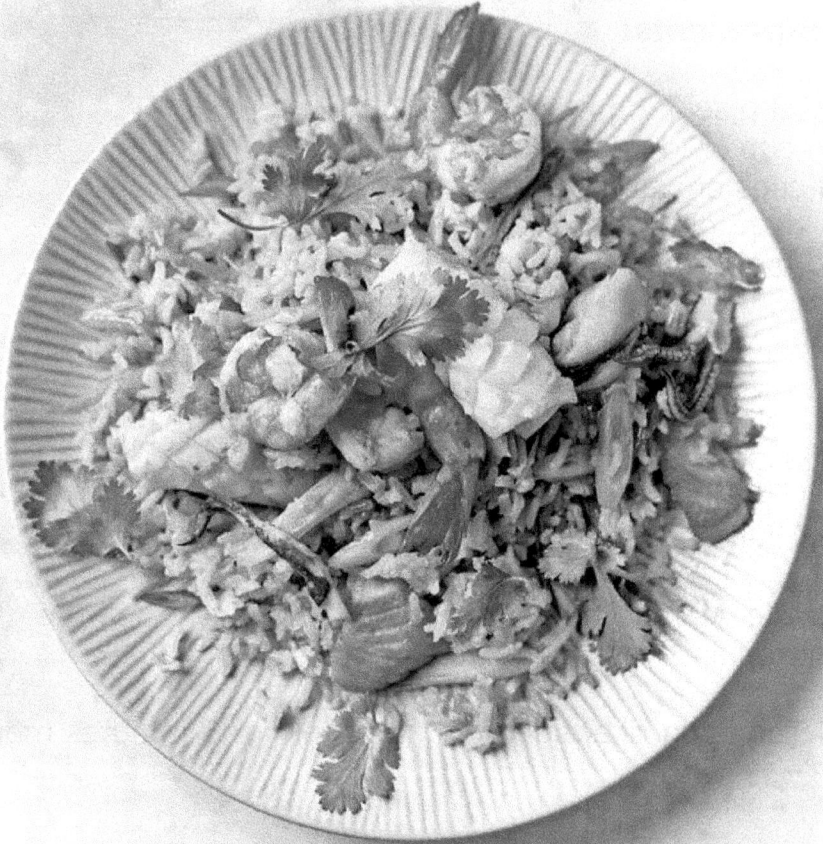

Vegetarian Pilaf
Preparation Time: 10 minutes
Cooking Time: 30 minutes
Servings: 6

Ingredients:

1 cup of long grain rice
2 cups of water
1 carrot, grated
2 tbsp. olive oil
1 tbsp. dried dill
½ tsp. dried mint
½ tsp. salt

Directions:

1.Boil rice with water for 15 minutes on medium heat.

2.Meanwhile, melt the olive oil and add the carrot.

3.Roast the carrot for 10 minutes or until it is soft.

4.Then add dried dill, mint, and cooked rice.

5.Carefully stir the pilaf and cook for 5 minutes.

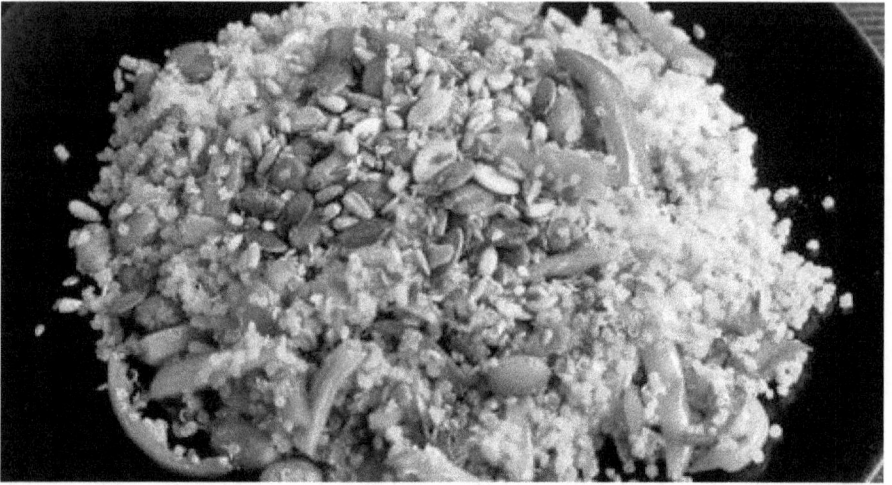

Creamy Garlic-Parmesan Chicken Pasta

Preparation Time: 5 minutes
Cooking Time: 25 minutes
Servings: 6

Ingredients:

2 boneless, skinless chicken breasts
3 tbsp. extra-virgin olive oil
1½ tsp. salt
1 large onion, thinly sliced
3 tbsp. garlic, minced
1 lb. fettuccine pasta
1 cup heavy (whipping) cream
¾ cup freshly grated Parmesan cheese, divided
½ tsp. freshly ground black pepper

Directions:

1.Bring a large pot of salted water to a simmer.

2.Cut the chicken into thin strips.

3.In a large skillet over medium heat, cook the olive oil and chicken for 3 minutes.

4.Next add the salt, onion, and garlic to the pan with the chicken. Cook for 7 minutes.

5.Bring the pot of salted water to a boil, add the pasta, and then cook for 7 minutes.

6.While the pasta is cooking, add the cream, ½ cup of Parmesan cheese, and black pepper to the chicken; simmer for 3 minutes.

7.Reserve ½ cup of the pasta water. Drain the pasta and add it to the chicken cream sauce.

8.Add the reserved pasta water to the pasta and toss together. Let simmer for 2 minutes. Top with the remaining ¼ cup Parmesan cheese and serve warm.

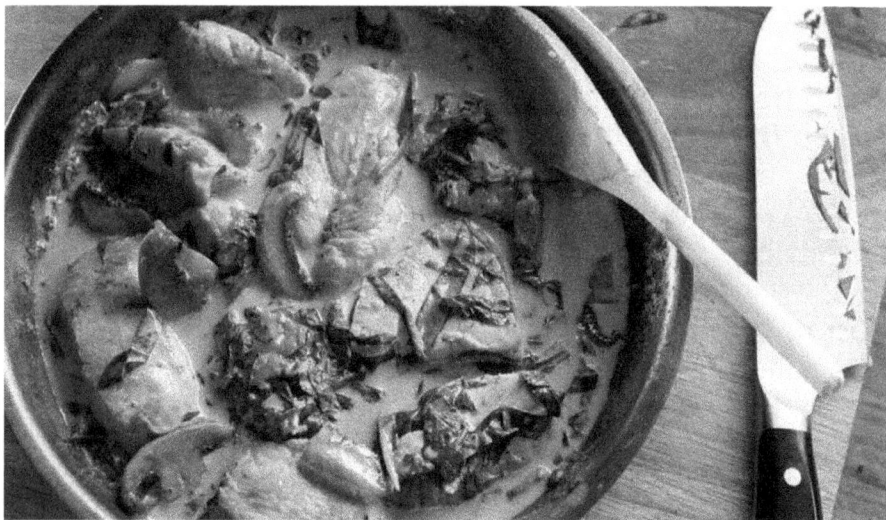

Artichoke Chicken Pasta
Preparation Time: 20 minutes
Cooking Time: 5 minutes
Servings: 4

Ingredients:

2 cloves garlic, crushed
2 lemons, wedged
2 tbsp. lemon juice
14 oz. artichoke hearts, chopped
1-lb. chicken breast fillet, diced
½ cup feta cheese, crumbled
1 tbsp. olive oil
16 oz. whole-wheat (gluten-free) pasta of your choice
3 tbsp. parsley, chopped
½ cup red onion, chopped
2 tsp. oregano
1 tomato, chopped Ground black pepper and salt, to taste

Directions:

1.Pour the water into a deep saucepan and boil it. Add the pasta and some salt; cook it as per package directions. Drain the water and set aside the pasta.

2.Over medium stove flame, heat the oil in a skillet or saucepan (preferably of medium size).

3.Sauté the onions and garlic until softened and translucent, stir in between.

4.Add the chicken and cook until it is no longer pink.

5.Mix in the tomatoes, artichoke hearts, parsley, feta cheese, oregano, lemon juice and the cooked pasta.

6.Combine well and cook for 3-4 minutes, stirring frequently.

7.Season with black pepper and salt. Garnish with lemon wedges and serve warm.

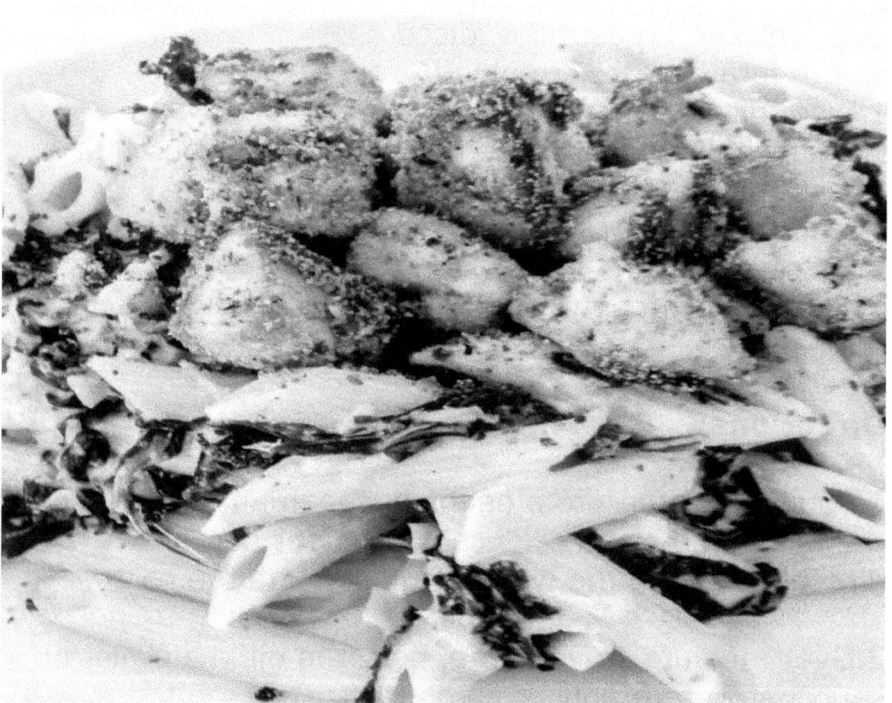

Spinach Beef Pasta

Preparation Time: 30 minutes
Cooking Time: 10 minutes
Servings: 4

Ingredients:

1 ¼ cups uncooked orzo pasta
¾ cup baby spinach
2 tbsp. olive oil
1 ½ lb. beef tenderloin
¾ cup feta cheese
2 quarts water
1 cup cherry tomatoes, halved
¼ tsp. salt

Directions:

1.Rub the meat with pepper and cut into small cubes.

2.Over medium stove flame; heat the oil in a deep saucepan (preferably of medium size).

3.Add and stir-fry the meat until it is evenly brown.

4.Add the water and boil the mixture; stir in the orzo and salt.

5.Cook the mixture for 7-8 minutes. Add the spinach and cook until it wilts.

6.Add the tomatoes and cheese; combine and serve warm.

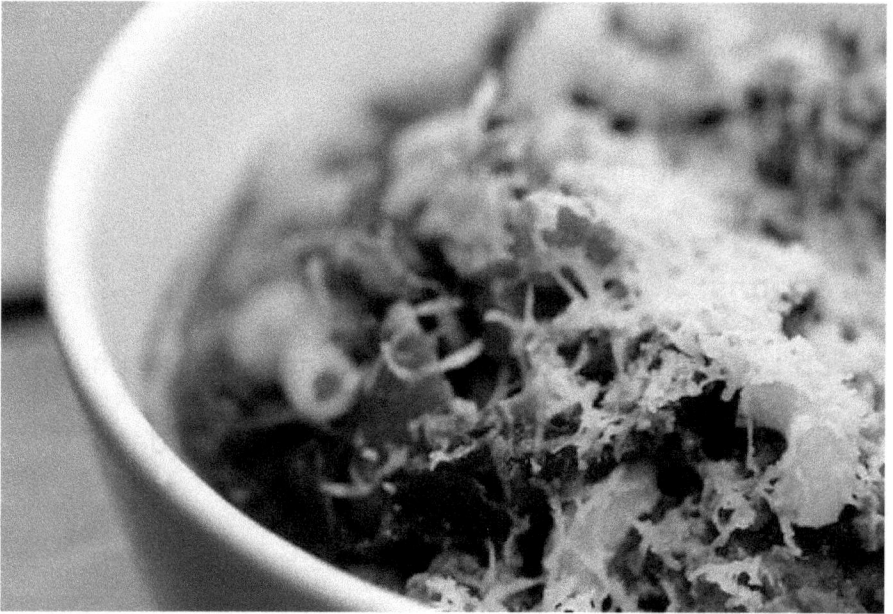

Asparagus Parmesan Pasta

Preparation Time: 25 minutes
Cooking Time: 4 minutes
Servings: 2

Ingredients:

1 tsp. extra-virgin olive oil
1 tsp. lemon juice
¾ cup whole milk
½ bunch asparagus, trimmed and cut into small pieces
½ cup parmesan cheese, grated
2 tbsp. garlic, minced
2 tbsp. almond flour
2 tsp. whole grain mustard
4 oz. whole-wheat penne pasta
1 tsp. tarragon, minced
Ground black pepper and salt, to taste

Directions:

1.Pour the water into a wide saucepan and boil it. Add the pasta and some salt; cook it as per package directions. Drain the water and set aside the pasta.

2.Take another pan, pour 8 cups of water and let it come to boiling. Add the asparagus and boil until it is soft. Drain and set aside.

3.In a mixing bowl, combine the milk, flour, mustard, black pepper and salt. Set aside.

4.Over medium stove flame, heat the oil in a skillet or saucepan (preferably of medium size).

5.Sauté the garlic until softened and fragrant, stirring in between.

6.Add the milk mixture and let it simmer. Add the tarragon, lemon juice and lemon zest; mix to combine.

7.Add the cooked pasta, asparagus, and simmer until the sauce thickens, stirring frequently.

8.Top with parmesan cheese and serve warm.

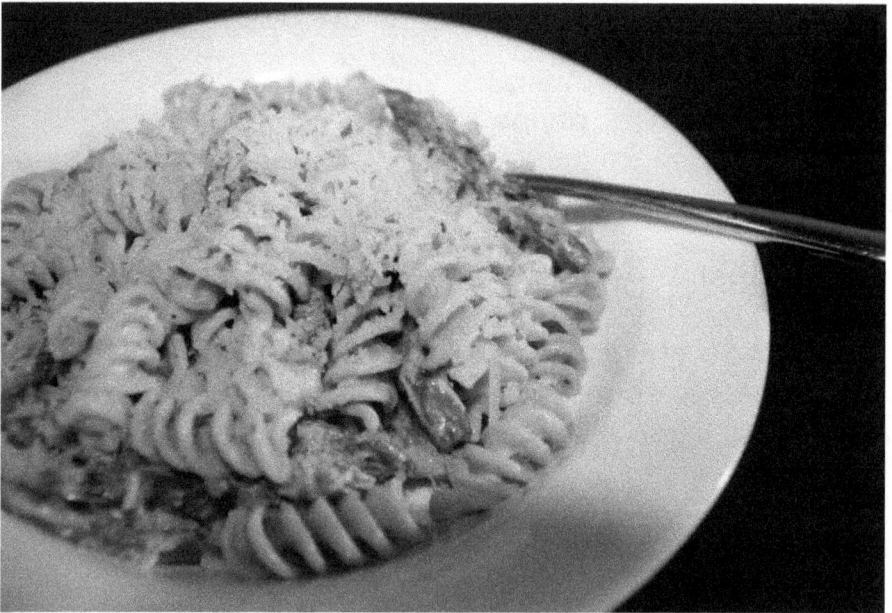

Mussels Linguine Delight

Preparation Time: 20 minutes
Cooking Time: 10 minutes
Servings: 4

Ingredients:

1 lb. mussels, cleaned and debearded
1 tbsp. olive oil
½ tsp. oregano
½ tsp. basil, chopped
1 clove garlic, minced
1 lemon, wedges
8 oz. whole-wheat linguine pasta
1 pinch pepper flakes, crushed
1 (14.5 oz.) can tomatoes, crushed
¼ cup white wine

Directions:

1.Pour the water into a deep saucepan and boil it. Add the pasta and some salt; cook it as per package directions. Drain the water and set aside the pasta.

2. Over a medium stove flame; heat the oil in a skillet or saucepan (preferably medium size).

3.Sauté the garlic until softened and fragrant, stir in between.

4.Add the tomatoes, basil, pepper flakes and oregano. Reduce the heat and simmer the mix.

5.Add the mussels, wine and increase the heat. Cook for 3-5 minutes.

6.Wait for the mussels to cook and open. Mix in the pasta.

7.Garnish with the parsley; serve with some lemon wedges on the side.

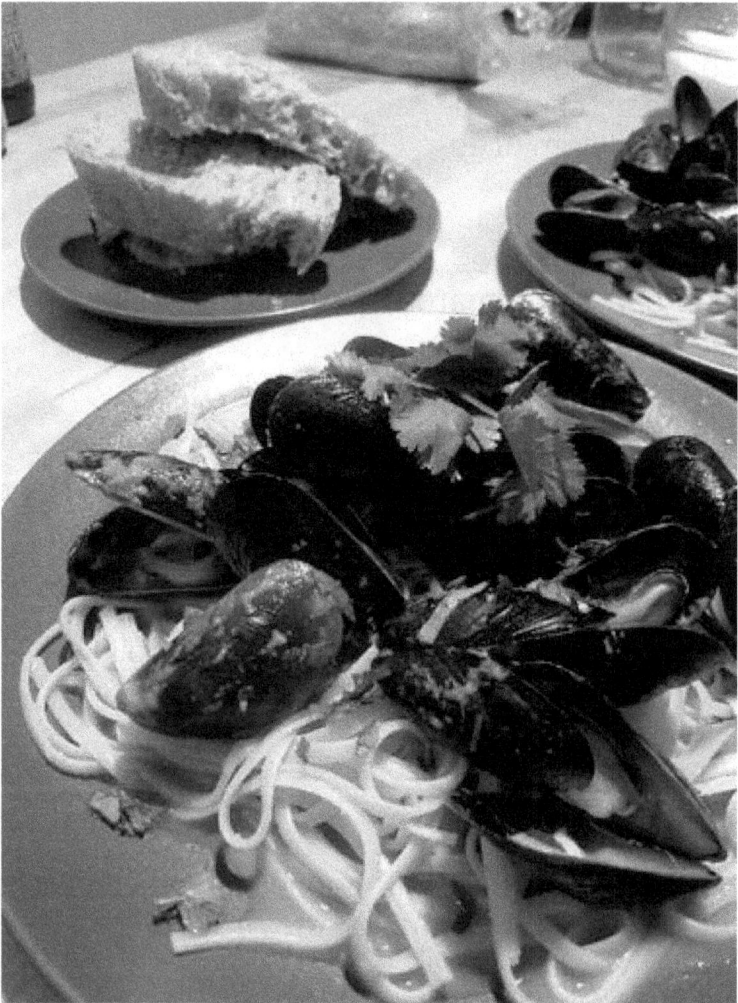

Arugula Pasta Soup

Preparation Time: 15 minutes
Cooking Time: 5 minutes
Servings: 6

Ingredients:

7 oz. chickpeas, rinsed
4 eggs, lightly beaten
2 tbsp. lemon juice
3 cups arugula, chopped
6 tbsp. parmesan cheese
6 cups chicken broth
1 pinch of nutmeg
1 bunch scallions, sliced (greens and whites sliced separately)
1 1/3 cups whole-wheat pasta shell
2 cups water
Ground black pepper, to taste

Directions:

1.In a cooking pot or deep saucepan, combine the pasta, scallion whites, chickpeas, water, broth and nutmeg.

2.Heat the mixture; cover and bring to a boil.

3.Take off the lid and simmer the mixture for about 4 minutes. Add the arugula and cook until it is wilted.

4.Mix in the eggs and season with black pepper and salt.

5.Mix in the lemon juice and scallion greens. Top with the parmesan cheese; serve warm.

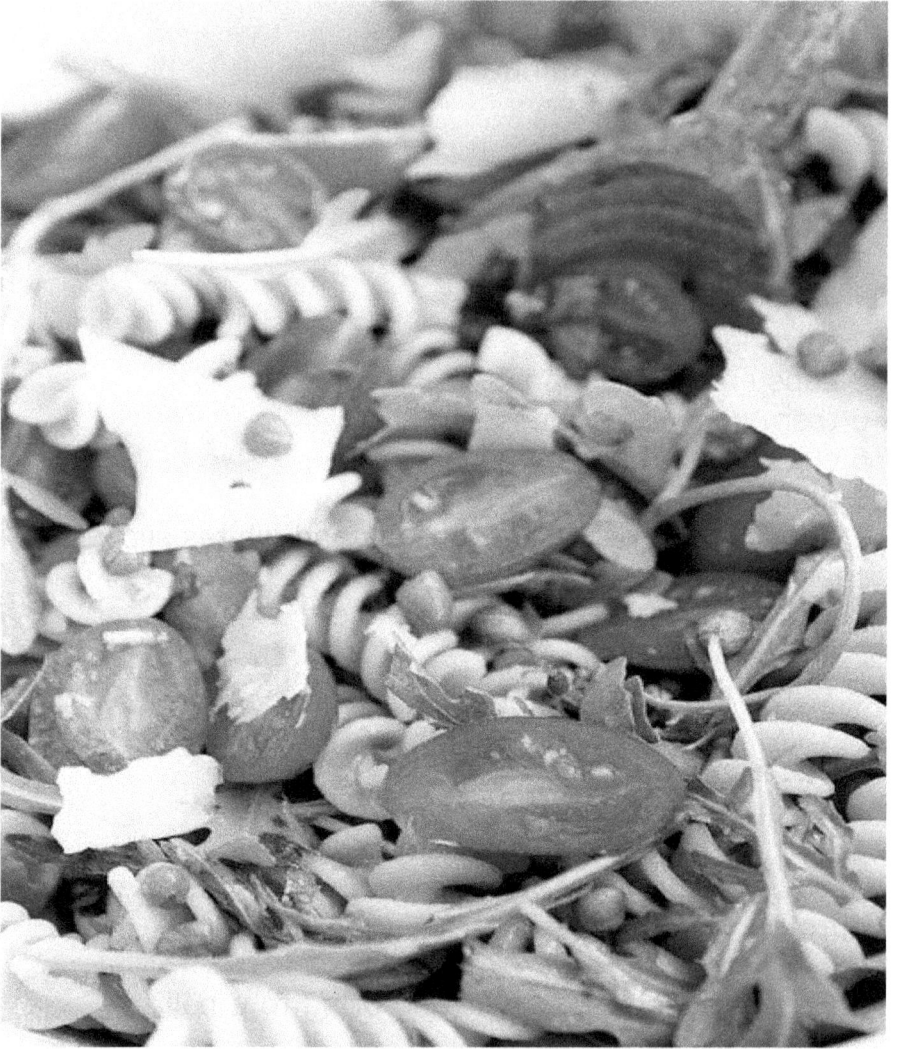

Pasta with garlic and Hoat Pepper
Preparation Time: 25 minutes
Cooking Time: 4 minutes
Servings: 4

Ingredients:

400g Spaghetti
8 tbsp. Extra virgin olive oil
4 cloves garlic, chopped
1 Chili pepper Coarse salt

Directions:

1.Put the water to boil, when it comes to a boil add salt and dip the spaghetti.

2.Meanwhile, in a saucepan heat the oil with the garlic deprived of the inner and chopped germ and the chopped peppers. Be careful: the flame should be sweet and the garlic should not darken.

3.Halfway through cooking, remove the spaghetti and continue cooking in the pan with the oil and garlic, adding the cooking water as if it were a risotto.

4.When cooked, serve the spaghetti.

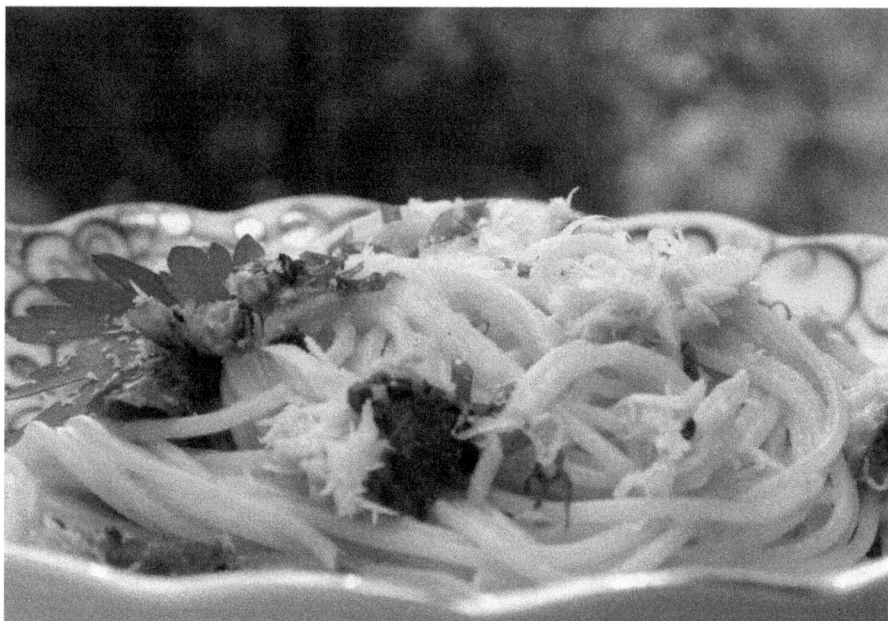

Stuffed Pasta Shells
Preparation Time: 15 minutes
Cooking Time: 10 minutes
Servings: 4

Ingredients:

5 Cups Marinara Sauce
15 Oz. Ricotta Cheese
1 ½ Cups Mozzarella Cheese, Grated
¾ Cup Parmesan Cheese, Grated
2 tbsp. Parsley, Fresh & Chopped
¼ Cup Basil Leaves, Fresh & Chopped
8 Oz. Spinach, Fresh & Chopped
½ tsp. Thyme
Sea Salt & Black Pepper to Taste
1 lb. Ground Beef
1 Cup Onions, Chopped
4 Cloves Garlic, Diced
2 tbsp. Olive Oil, Divided
12 Oz. Jumbo Pasta Shells

Directions:

1.Start by cooking your pasta shells by following your package instructions. Once they're cooked, then set them to the side.

2.Press sauté and then add in half of your olive oil. Cook your garlic and onions, which should take about four minutes. Your onions should be tender, and your garlic should be fragrant.

3.Add your ground beef in, seasoning it with thyme, salt, and pepper, cooking for another four minutes.

4.Add in your basil, pa

rsley, spinach and marinara sauce.

5.Cover your pot, and cook for five minutes on low pressure.

6.Use a quick release, and top with cheeses.

7.Press sauté again, making sure that it stays warm until your cheese melts.

8.Take a tbsp. of the mixture, stuffing it into your pasta shells.

9.Top with your remaining sauce before serving warm.

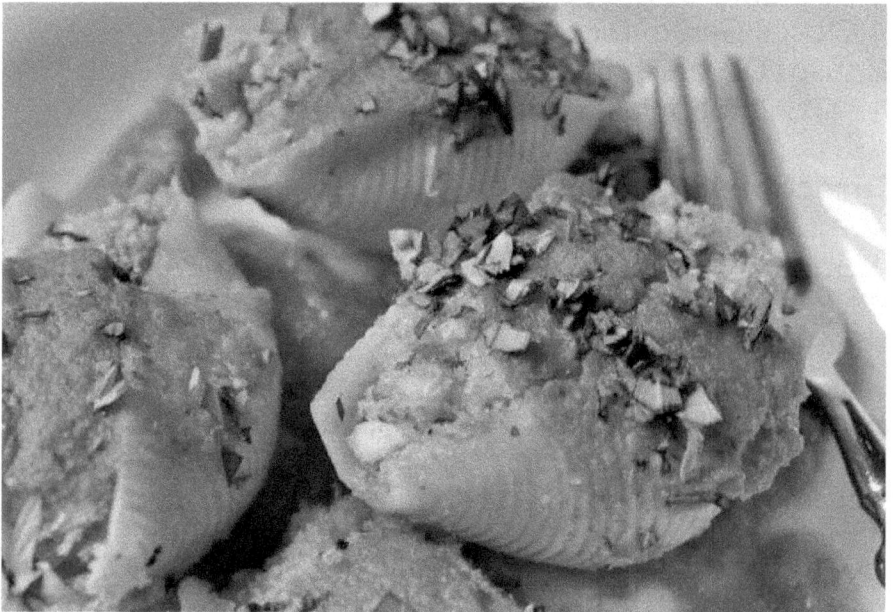

Homemade Pasta Bolognese

Preparation Time: 20 minutes
Cooking Time: 10 minutes
Servings: 4

Ingredients:

17 oz. Minced meat.
12 oz. Pasta
1 piece Sweet red onion
2 cloves Garlic
1 tbsp Vegetable oil
3 tbsp Tomato paste
2 oz. Grated Parmesan Cheese
3 pieces Bacon

Directions:

1.Fry finely chopped onions and garlic in a frying pan in vegetable oil until a characteristic smell.

2.Add minced meat and chopped bacon to the pan. Constantly break the lumps with a spatula and mix so that the minced meat is crumbly.

3.When the mince is ready, add tomato paste, grated Parmesan to the pan, mix, reduce heat and leave to simmer.

4.At this time, boil the pasta. I don't salt water because tomato paste and sauce turn out to be quite salty for me.

5.When the pasta is ready, discard it in a colander, arrange it on plates, add meat sauce with tomato paste on top of each serving.

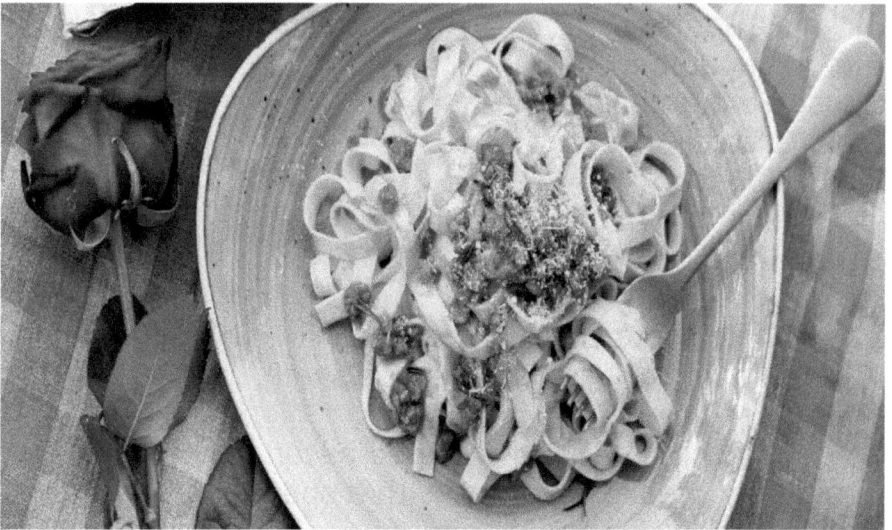

Asparagus Pasta

Preparation Time: 10 minutes
Cooking Time: 25 Minutes
Servings: 6

Ingredients:

8 Oz. Farfalle Pasta, Uncooked
1 ½ Cups Asparagus, Fresh, Trimmed & Chopped into 1 Inch Pieces
1 Pint Grape Tomatoes, Halved
2 tbsp. Olive Oil
Sea Salt & Black Pepper to Taste
2 Cups Mozzarella, Fresh & Drained
1/3 Cup Basil Leaves, Fresh & Torn
2 tbsp. Balsamic Vinegar

Directions:

1.Start by heating the oven to 400°F, and then get out a stockpot.

2. Cook your pasta per package instructions, and reserve ¼ cup of pasta water.

3.Get out a bowl and toss the tomatoes, oil, asparagus, and season with salt and pepper. Spread this mixture on a baking sheet, and bake for fifteen minutes. Stir twice in this time.

4.Remove your vegetables from the oven, and then add the cooked pasta to your baking sheet. Mix with a few tbsp. of pasta water so that your sauce becomes smoother.

5.Mix in your basil and mozzarella, drizzling with balsamic vinegar. Serve warm.

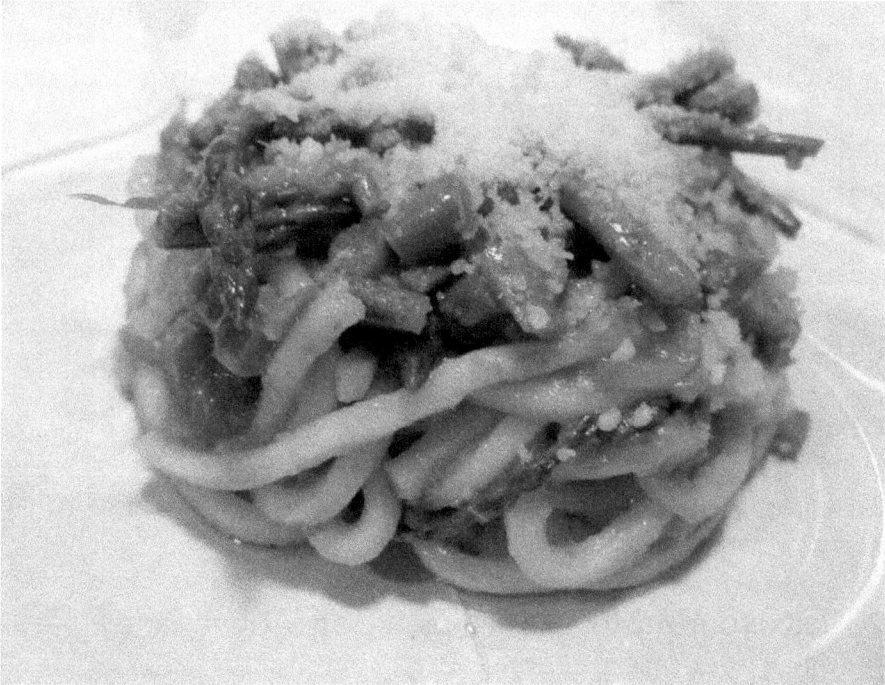

Penne Bolognese Pasta

Preparation Time: 15 minutes
Cooking Time: 20 minutes
Servings: 2

Ingredients:

7 oz. Penne pasta
5 oz Beef
1 oz. Parmesan Cheese
1 oz. Celery Stalk
26 g. Shallots
1,5 oz. Carrot
1 clove Garlic
1 g. Thyme
6 oz. Tomatoes in own juice
3 g. Parsley
1 g. Oregano
20 g. Butter
50 ml. Dry white wine
40 ml. Olive oil

Directions:

1.Pour the penne into boiling salted water and cook for 9 minutes.

2.Roll the beef through a meat grinder.

3.Dice onion, celery, carrots and garlic in a small cube.

4.Fry the chopped vegetables in a heated frying pan in olive oil with minced meat for 4–5 minutes, salt and pepper.

5.Add oregano to the fried minced meat and vegetables, pour 50 ml of wine, add the tomatoes along with the juice and simmer for 10 minutes until the tomatoes are completely softened.

6.Add the boiled penne and butter to the sauce and simmer for 1-2 minutes, stirring continuously.

7.Put in a plate, sprinkle with grated Parmesan and chopped parsley, decorate with a sprig of thyme and serve.

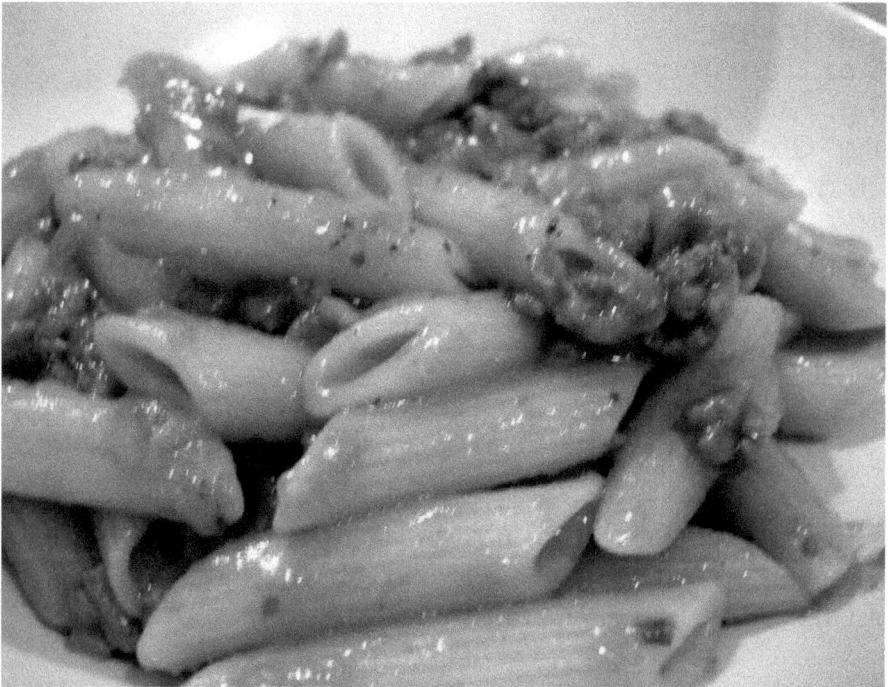

Quick Pasta Bolognese

Preparation Time: 10 minutes
Cooking Time: 25 minutes
Servings: 2

Ingredients:

17 oz. Ground beef
2 cloves. Garlic
3 tbsp. Tomato paste
14 oz. Tomatoes
150 ml. Beef broth
A mixture of Italian herbs 1 tsp.
14 oz. Penne pasta
Basil leaves to taste Fresh mushrooms to taste

Directions:

1.Prepare the paste following the instructions on the packaging.

2.Heat the oil in a pan, sauté the minced meat for 5 minutes, then add the mushrooms and fry for another 3 minutes.

3.Add garlic and tomato paste and simmer for 2 minutes.

4.Add tomatoes, broth or wine, dried herbs and spices. Bring to a boil and simmer for 10 minutes.

5.Drain the water from the pasta, mix it with the sauce, sprinkle with basil leaves on top.

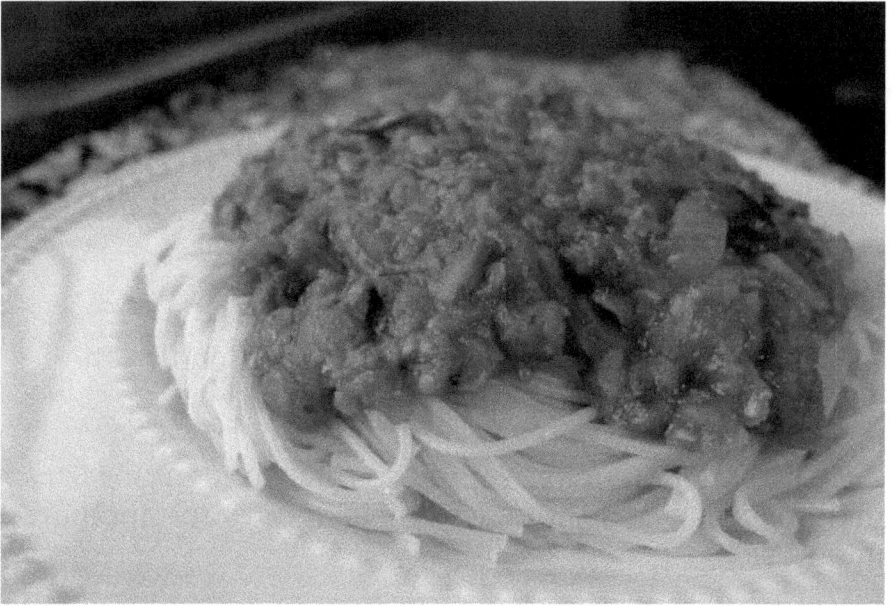

Pilaf with Cream Cheese

Preparation Time: 10 minutes
Cooking Time: 30 Minutes
Servings: 4

Ingredients:

2 Cups Yellow Long Grain Rice, Parboiled
1 Cup Onion
4 Green Onions
3 tbsp. Butter
3 tbsp. Vegetable Broth
2 tsp. Cayenne Pepper
1 tsp. Paprika
½ tsp. Cloves, Minced
2 tbsp. Mint Leaves, Fresh & Chopped
1 Bunch Fresh Mint Leaves to Garnish
1 tbsp. Olive Oil
Sea Salt & Black Pepper to Taste
3 tbsp. Olive Oil
Sea Salt & Black Pepper to Taste
9 Oz. Cream Cheese

Directions:

1.Start by heating your oven to 360°F, and then get out a pan. Heat your butter and olive oil together, and cook your onions and spring onions for two minutes.

2.Add in your salt, pepper, paprika, cloves, vegetable broth, rice and remaining seasoning. Sauté for three minutes.

3.Cover with foil, and bake for another half hour. Allow it to cool.

4.Mix in the cream cheese, cheese, olive oil, salt and pepper. Serve your pilaf garnished with fresh mint leaves.

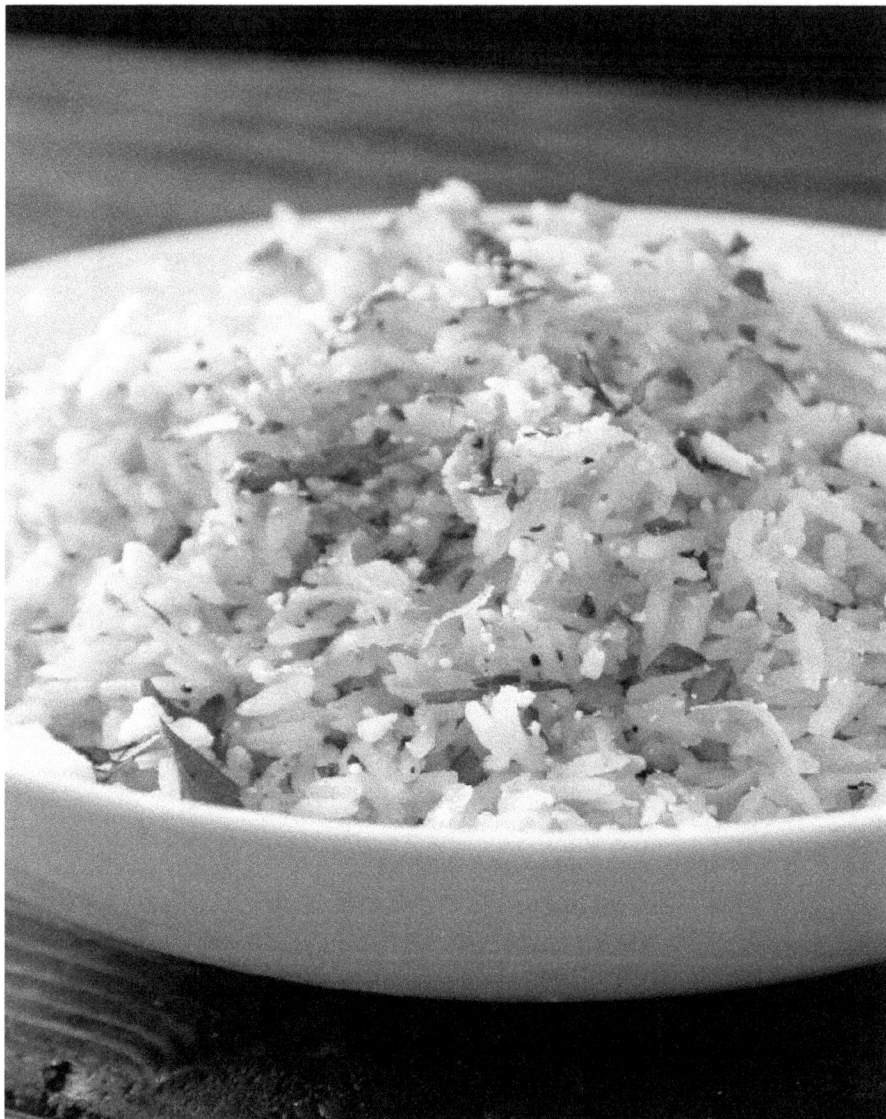

Herbed Pasta

Preparation Time: 15 minutes
Cooking Time: 15 minutes
Servings: 4

Ingredients:

1 (8-oz.) package linguini pasta
2 tbsp. olive oil
1 tbsp. garlic, minced
1 tbsp. dried oregano, crushed
1 tbsp. dried basil, crushed
1 tsp. dried thyme, crushed
2 cups plum tomatoes, chopped

Directions:

1.In a large pan of lightly salted boiling water, add the pasta and cook for about 8-10 minutes or according to package's directions.

2.Drain the pasta well.

3.In a large skillet, heat oil over medium heat and sauté the garlic for about 1 minute.

4.Stir in herbs and sauté for about 1 minute more.

5.Add the pasta and cook for about 2-3 minutes or until heated completely.

6.Fold in tomatoes and remove from heat. Serve hot.

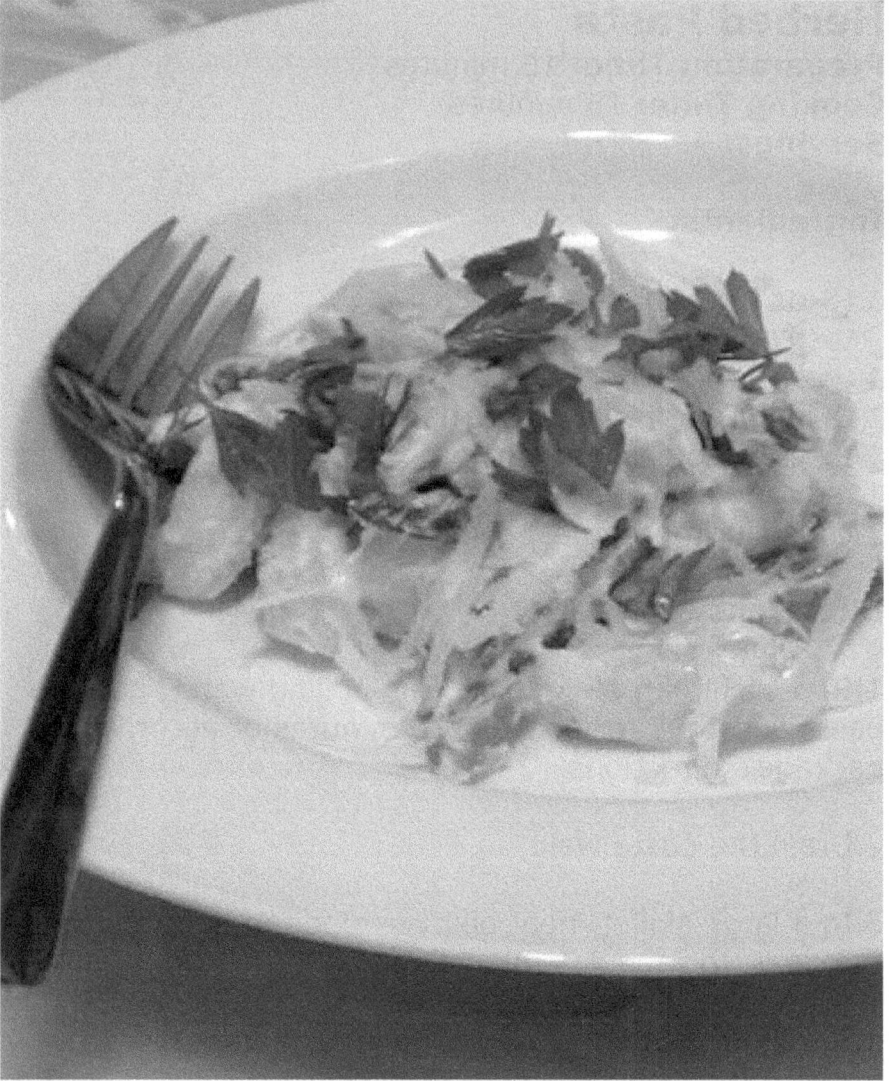

Pasta with Veggies

Preparation Time: 15 minutes
Cooking Time: 20 minutes
Servings: 6

Ingredients:

1 tomatoes
1-lb. farfalle pasta
¼ cup olive oil
1-lb. fresh mushrooms, sliced
3 garlic cloves, minced
1 tsp. dried oregano, crushed
1 (2-oz.) can black olives, drained
¾ cup feta cheese, crumbled

Directions:

1.In a large pan of the salted boiling water, add the tomatoes and cook for about 1 minute.

2.With a slotted spoon, transfer the tomatoes into a bowl of ice water.

3.In the same pan of the boiling water, add the pasta and cook for about 8-10 minutes.

4.Drain the pasta well.

5.Meanwhile, peel the blanched tomatoes and then chop them.

6.In a large skillet, heat oil over medium heat and sauté the mushrooms and garlic for about 4-5 minutes.

7.Add the tomatoes and oregano and cook for about 3-4 minutes.

8.Divide the pasta onto serving plates and top with mushroom mixture.

9.Garnish with olives and feta and serve.

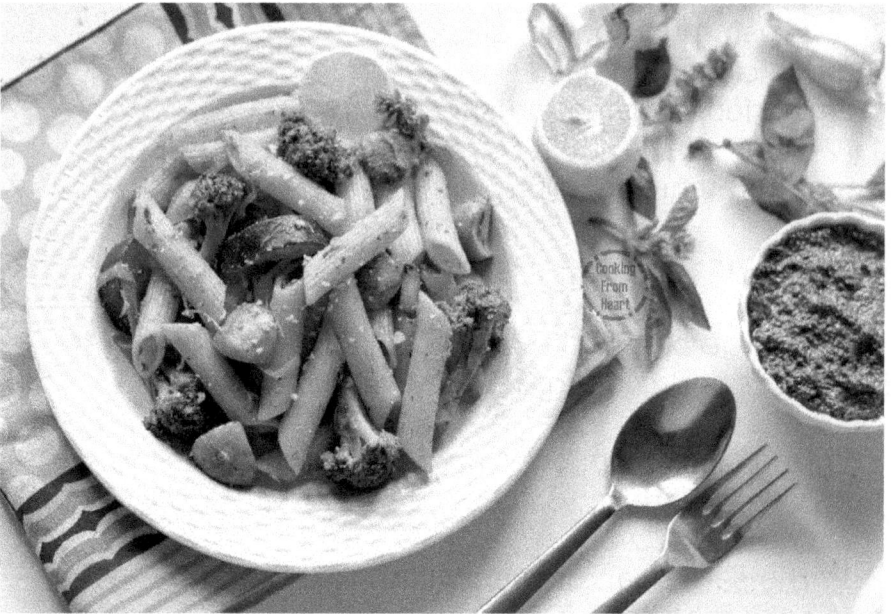

Pasta with Chicken & Veggies

Preparation Time: 15 minutes
Cooking Time: 10 minutes
Servings: 7

Ingredients:

3 tbsp. olive oil
1-lb. boneless, skinless chicken breast, sliced diagonally
1 (8½-oz.) jar sun-dried tomatoes, julienned
2 tbsp. garlic, minced
1-lb. angel hair pasta
1 (8½-oz.) can water-packed artichoke hearts,
quartered and drained
½ cup kalamata olive, pitted
¼ cup fresh basil
6 oz. feta cheese, crumbled
¼ cup heavy cream
1 tsp. dried oregano
Salt and ground black pepper, as required

Directions:

1.In a skillet, heat the oil over medium heat and sear the chicken strips for about 5-6 minutes or until browned completely.

2.Add the sun-dried tomatoes and garlic and sauté for about 2 minutes.

3.Meanwhile, in a large pan of the salted boiling water, add the pasta and cook for about 5-6 minutes.

4.Drain the pasta well.
In the skillet, add the artichoke hearts, olives, basil and feta cheese and sauté for about 1 minute.

5.Add the cream and stir to combine. Stir in the oregano, salt and black pepper and remove from the heat.

6.In a large serving bowl, add the pasta and chicken mixture and toss to coat well.

7.Serve immediately.

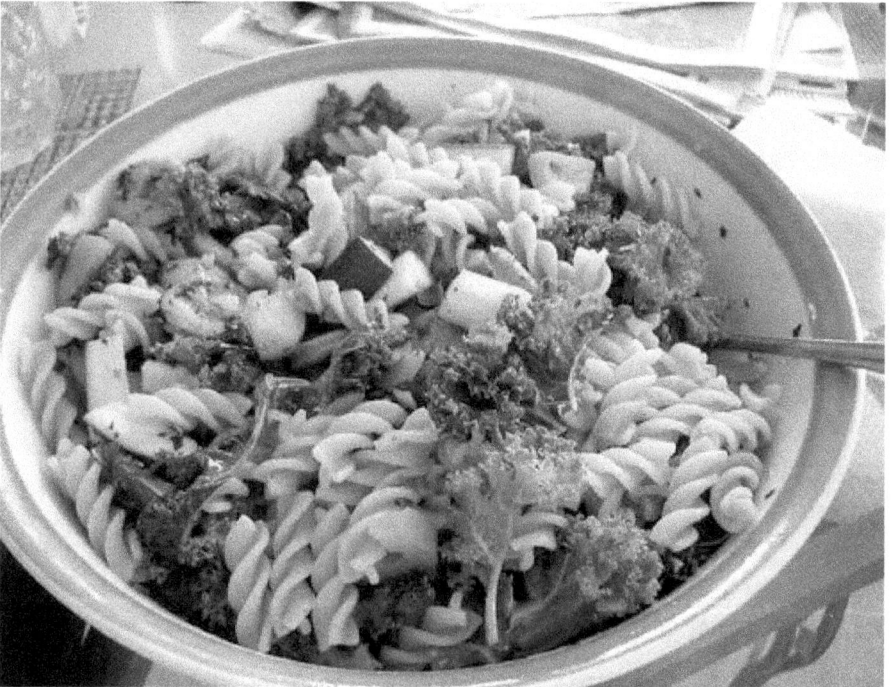

Pasta with Shrimp & Spinach

Preparation Time: 15 minutes
Cooking Time: 10 minutes
Servings: 4

Ingredients:

1 cup sour cream
½ cup feta cheese, crumbled
3 garlic cloves, chopped
2 tsp. dried basil, crushed
¼ tsp. red pepper flakes, crushed
8 oz. fettuccine pasta
1 (10-oz.) packages frozen spinach, thawed
12 oz. medium shrimp, peeled and deveined
Salt and ground black pepper, as required

Directions:

1. In a large serving bowl, add the sour cream, feta, garlic, basil, red pepper flakes, salt, and mix well.

2. Set aside until using.

3. In a large pan of the lightly salted boiling water, add the fettucine and cook for about 10 minutes or according to the package's directions.

4. After 8 minutes, stir in the spinach and shrimp and cook for about 2 minutes.

5. Drain the pasta mixture well.

6. Add the hot pasta mixture into the sour cream mixture and gently, toss to coat.

7.Serve immediately.

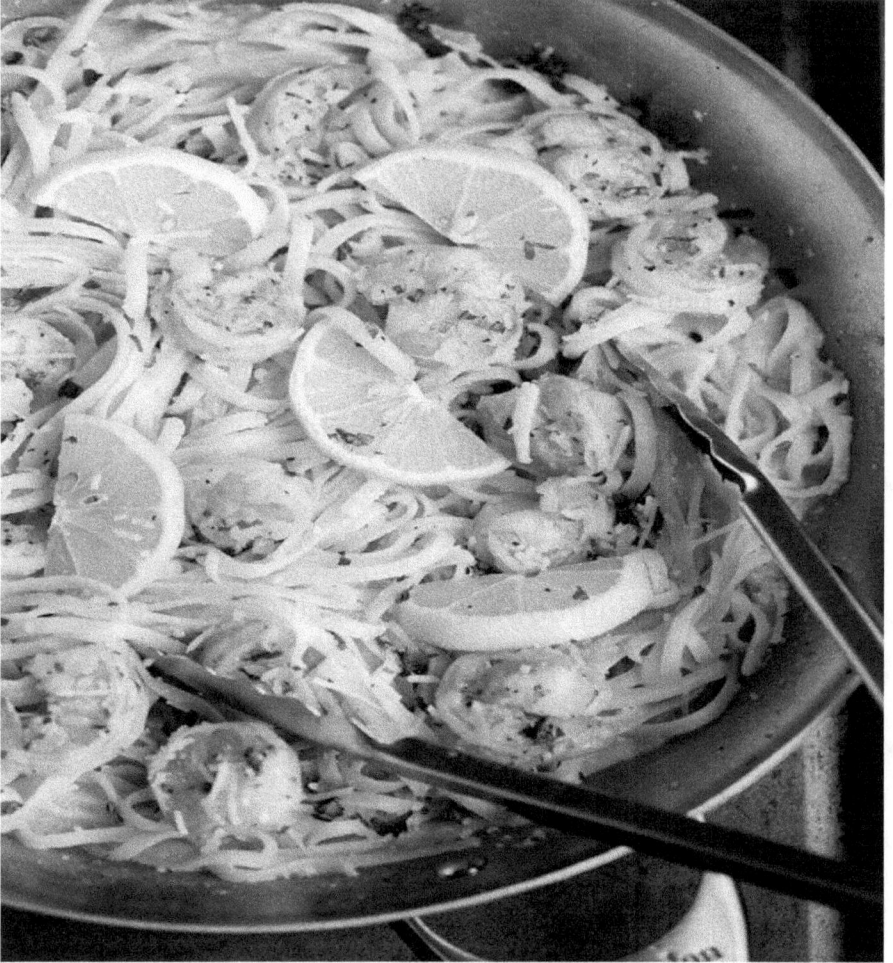

Carbonara Pasta With Champignons
Preparation Time: 10 minutes
Cooking Time: 25 minutes
Servings: 2

Ingredients:

9 oz. Spaghetti
7 oiz. Bacon
7 oz. Cream 20%
3,5 oz. Parmesan Cheese
4 pieces Egg yolk
5 cloves Garlic
5 oz. Champignons.
10 ml. Olive oil
Salt to taste
Ground black pepper to taste

Directions:

1.Prepare the ingredients.

2.Cut the bacon into strips, chop the garlic finely, chop the mushrooms.

3.Fry the garlic in a pan, then the mushrooms and bacon.

4.Grate the parmesan.

5.Put egg yolks in a plate, salt, pepper and beat.

6.Add cream and grated cheese to the yolks, mix.

7.Boil spaghetti to al dente (about a minute less than indicated on the packet).

8.Put the spaghetti in a pan, add the sauce, bacon and mushrooms.

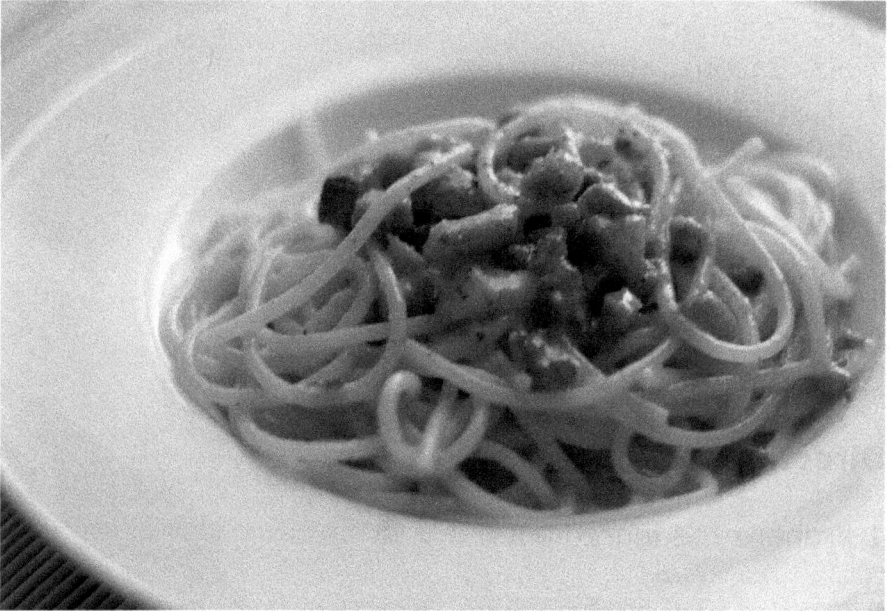

Spaghetti Carbonara With Red Onion

Preparation Time: 15 minutes
Cooking Time: 25 minutes
Servings: 4

Ingredients:

9 oz. Spaghetti.
3/4oz. Butter.
2 cloves Garlic
1 head Red onion
2 oz. Bacon
200ml. Cream 20%
2 oz. Grated Parmesan Cheese
4 eggs
Salt to taste
Ground black pepper to taste

Directions:

1.Boil water in a large saucepan and cook the pasta until al dente. Usually for this you need to cook it for a minute less than indicated on the pack.

2.While the pasta is boiling, melt the butter in a pan and fry finely chopped onion, garlic and bacon on it. To softness and a distinct garlic and fried bacon smell.

3.Remove the pan from the heat and beat four egg yolks with cream and grated Parmesan in a deep bowl. Salt and pepper the mixture, whisk again.

4.In the prepared spaghetti, pour the pieces of bacon fried with onions and garlic. Pour in a mixture of cream, yolks and parmesan, mix. And serve immediately, sprinkled with freshly grated cheese and black pepper

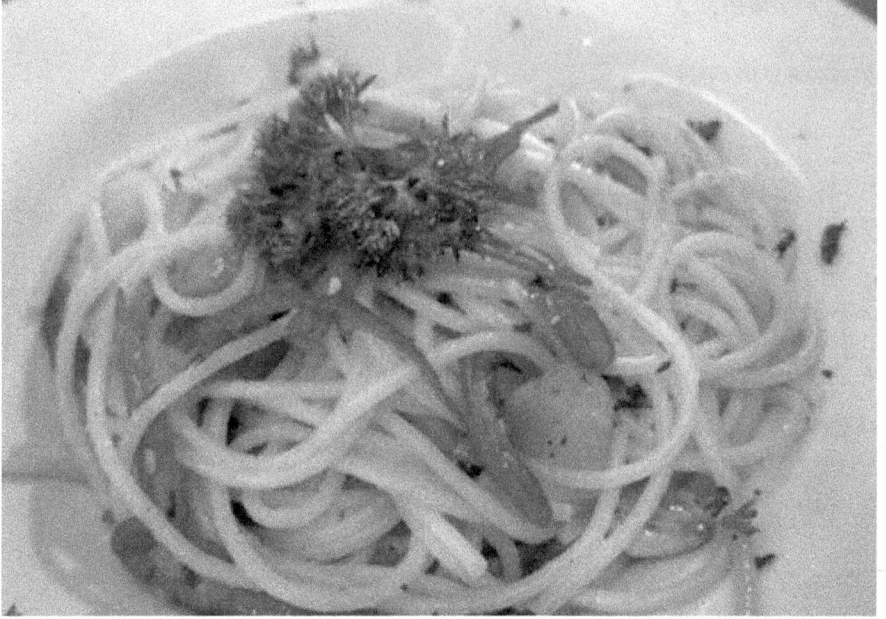

Cuttlefish Pasta With Carbonara Sauce

Preparation Time: 15 minutes
Cooking Time: 30 minutes
Servings: 3

Ingredients:

7 oz. Pasta
5 oz. Smoked bacon
2 oz. Grated Parmesan Cheese
7 oz. Champignons
200 ml. Cream
1 piece Egg yolk
3 cloves Garlic
2 tbsp Butter
Ground black pepper pinch Ground nutmeg pinch

Directions:

1.Boil spaghetti. At this time, fry the garlic and bacon in butter for three minutes.

2.Add the mushroom slices to the bacon, mix and fry for eight to ten minutes. During this time, the spaghetti will cook, drain from them and add to the mushrooms and bacon.

3.The final stage - cream, egg yolk, ground black pepper, ground nutmeg and grated cheese. Beat all this and pour spaghetti, fry for five minutes and serve.

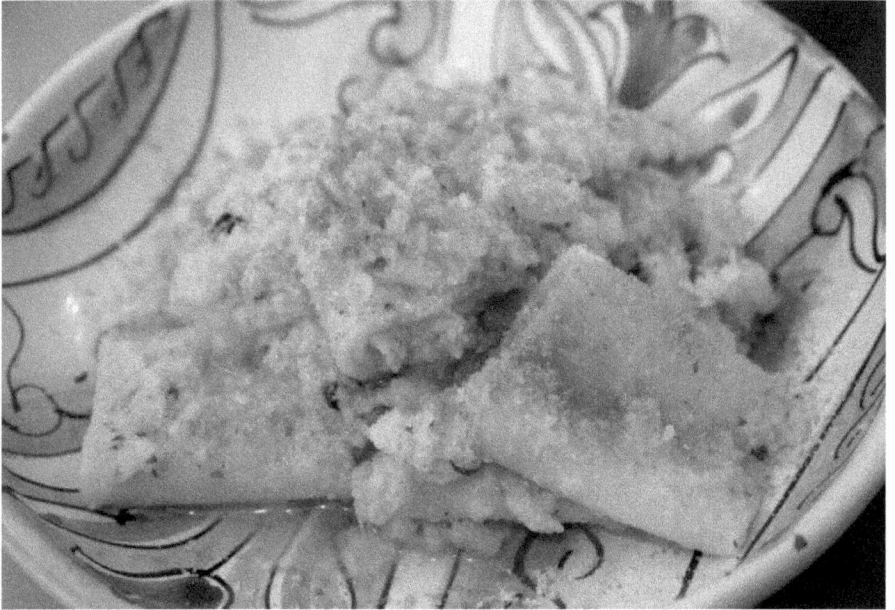

Spaghetti Carbonara
Preparation Time: 10 minutes
Cooking Time: 25 minutes
Servings: 2

Ingredients:

160 g. Spaghetti
4 oz. Pancetta
2 oz. Hard cheese
2 pieces Egg yolk
Salt to taste
Freshly ground black pepper to taste

Directions:

1.Bring well-salted water to a boil. Cook spaghetti to al dente. Save a little broth from the paste; you may need it. Drain the rest.

2.While preparing the pasta, heat the pan and fry the pancetta until golden, remove from heat.

3.In a small bowl, beat the yolks with grated cheese until smooth.

4.Return the pan with the pancetta to a small fire, add about 50 ml of the broth from the pasta, throw the spaghetti there and mix well until the boiling stops. Most of the water should boil.

5.Remove the pan from the heat and add the yolks with cheese and mix quickly until the yolks thicken. If the sauce seems too thick, add a little more paste broth. Pepper and salt to taste, serve.

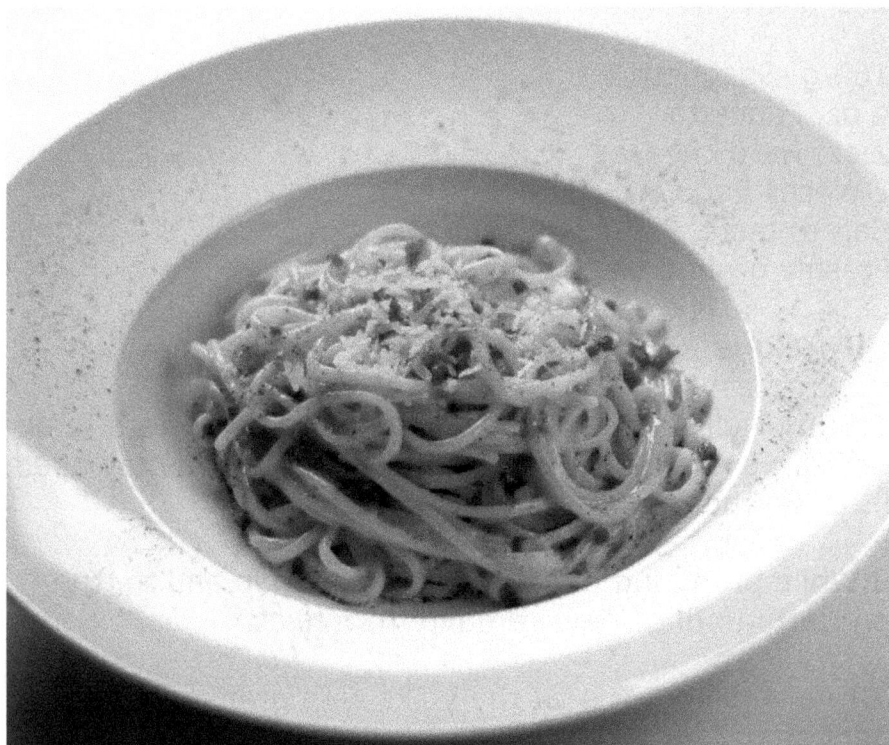

Chanterelle Pasta

Preparation Time: 15 minutes
Cooking Time: 30 minutes
Servings: 4

Ingredients:

7oz. Chanterelles Tagliatelle pasta
7 oz. Tomato Sauce
2 cloves Garlic
20 ml. Olive oil
30 ml. Dry white wine
10 g. Butter
2 oz. Parmesan Cheese
Salt to taste
Ground black pepper to taste

Directions:

1.Heat olive oil in a pan with a thick bottom, add a couple of whole cloves of garlic, add chanterelles (pre-washed and well- dried).

2.Fry the chanterelles 5-7 minutes until golden brown, pour in white wine, evaporate.

3.Then pour the tomato sauce and simmer for about 5 minutes. At the end, add butter, salt and pepper.

4.Add the paste cooked al-dente to the sauce and mix. Serve garnished with sliced parmesan and parsley.

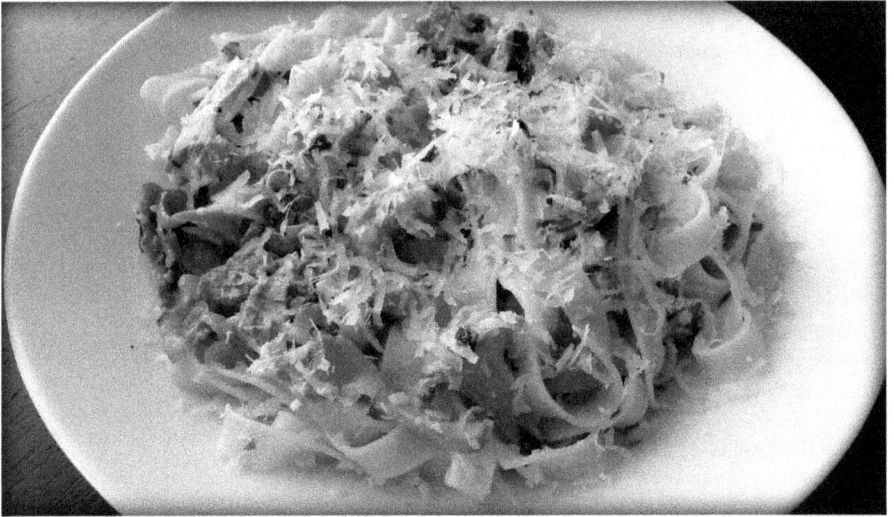

Pasta "Verochka"

Preparation Time: 5 minutes
Cooking Time: 20 minutes
Servings: 2

Ingredients:

10 oz. Spaghetti
200 ml. Cream 33%
3,5 oz. Lightly salted trout
2 oz. Grated Parmesan Cheese
Dried oregano to taste
Dried basil to taste

Directions:

1.Boil spaghetti - or other suitable pasta - until cooked, following the time indicated on the package. You do not need to salt water - the salt will give the fish.

2.Meanwhile, finely chop the red fish - not necessarily trout, any. And its quantity may be different - if only the fish had no more pasta.

3.Heat the cream in a pan (it is better to take Fatter) and add fish. Keep on fire, stirring constantly and, most importantly, not boiling. When the fish loses color, you can remove the pan from the heat.

4.Throw the prepared pasta into a colander and add to the sauce. Or add the sauce to the paste - as anyone is more familiar and convenient. Add oregano and basil, mix.

5.Sprinkle the paste spread on the plates with grated Parmesan.

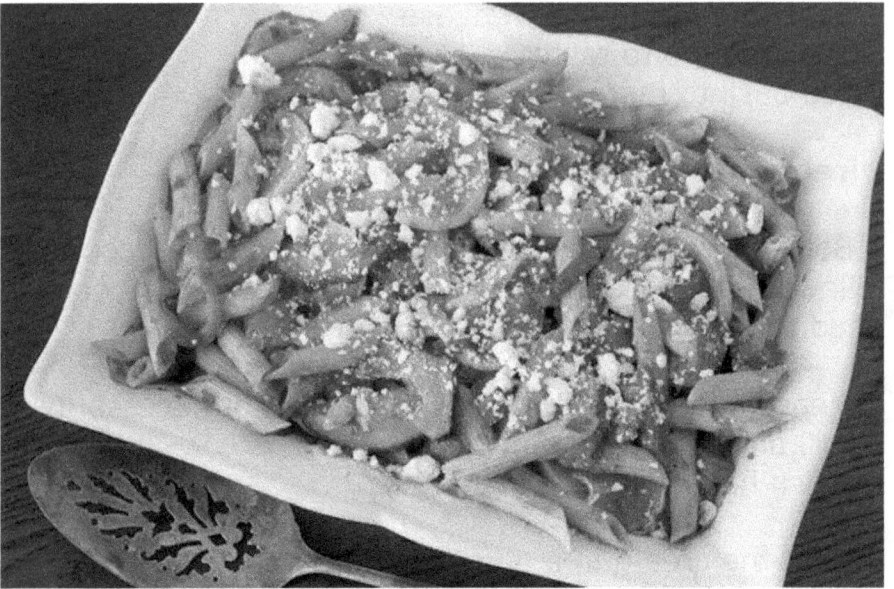

Pasta e Patate
Preparation Time: 15 minutes
Cooking Time: 30 minutes
Servings: 3

Ingredients:

5 oz. Bacon
3 oz. Onions
8 oz. Spaghetti.
14 oz. Potato
3 oz. Parmesan Cheese
30 ml. Olive oil
Freshly ground black pepper to taste
Salt to taste

Directions:

1.Fry the bacon in a dry skillet. Add olive oil and fry finely chopped onions, not until golden brown.

2.Add chopped potatoes to the onion, fry and add water to the onion. Cook until al dente, 5-10 minutes.

3.Break the spaghetti, toss it to the potatoes, add water, continue cooking until the spaghetti is ready. Pour a little water over the entire cooking process so that a little liquid is left in the finale, sufficient to make a sauce.

4.In the finale add grated parmesan, olive oil, freshly ground black pepper, mix well

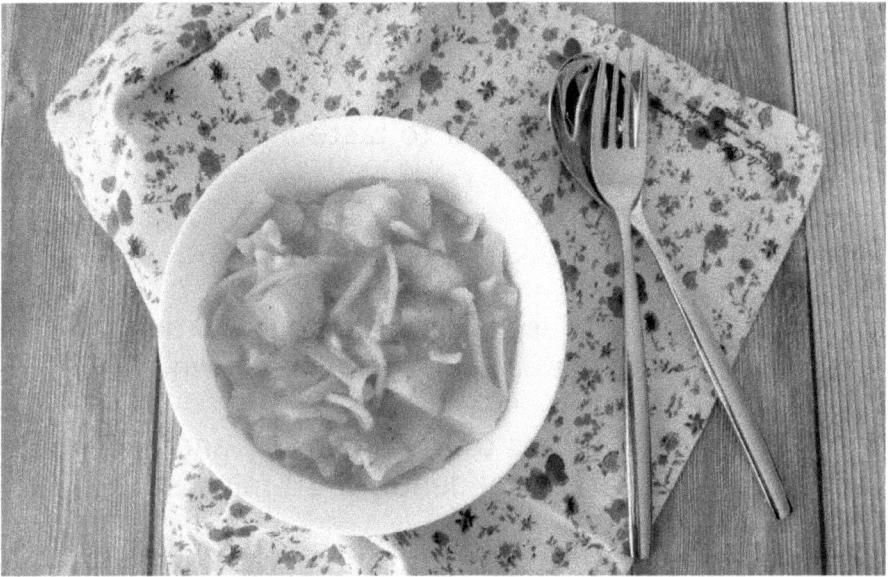

Pasta with Fresh Tomatoes

Preparation Time: 15 minutes
Cooking Time: 30 minutes
Servings: 3

Ingredients:

7 oz. Tagliatelle pasta
1 piece Tomatoes
5 black olives
Garlic 2 cloves Olive oil 50 ml

Directions:

1.Boil the pasta in salted boiling water.

2.Simultaneously in 1 tbsp. of olive oil, lightly fry the garlic and sliced olives.

3.Dice the fresh tomatoes and add to the garlic and olives. Cooking tomatoes is not necessary, they should only warm up.

4.Slightly salt and pepper the sauce.

5.Drain the water and combine the pasta with the sauce.

6.Put the pasta in a plate and lightly pour olive oil.

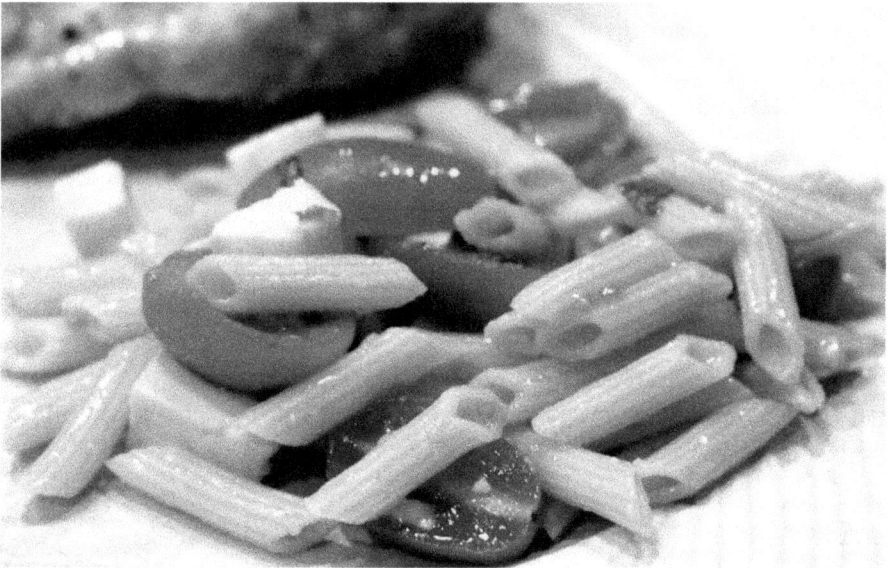

Spaghetti Carbonara With Chicken

Preparation Time: 5 minutes
Cooking Time: 30 minutes
Servings: 2

Ingredients:

10 oz. Durum wheat spaghetti
100 ml. Cream
2 cloves Garlic 2
3 Chicken egg
Basil to taste
15 g. Sesame seeds
Salt to taste
3 tbsp. Olive oil
2 oz. Parmesan Cheese
7 oz. Chicken fillet

Directions:

1.Finely chop the chicken fillet and fry in olive oil until tender.

2.Peel the garlic, chop finely and add to the chicken. Fry it all together for 1-2 minutes. Then add cream, salt to taste. Stew on low heat so that the cream does not curl.

3.Add a spoonful of olive oil to boiling water, salt to taste to taste. Cooking spaghetti to al dente.

4.Cooking the sauce. To do this, beat the eggs, then add basil, salt, sesame and grated parmesan.

5.Once the spaghetti is ready, we discard them in a colander, then - in a pan with chicken and garlic, pour everything in the resulting sauce and simmer for another 2-3 minutes over low heat.

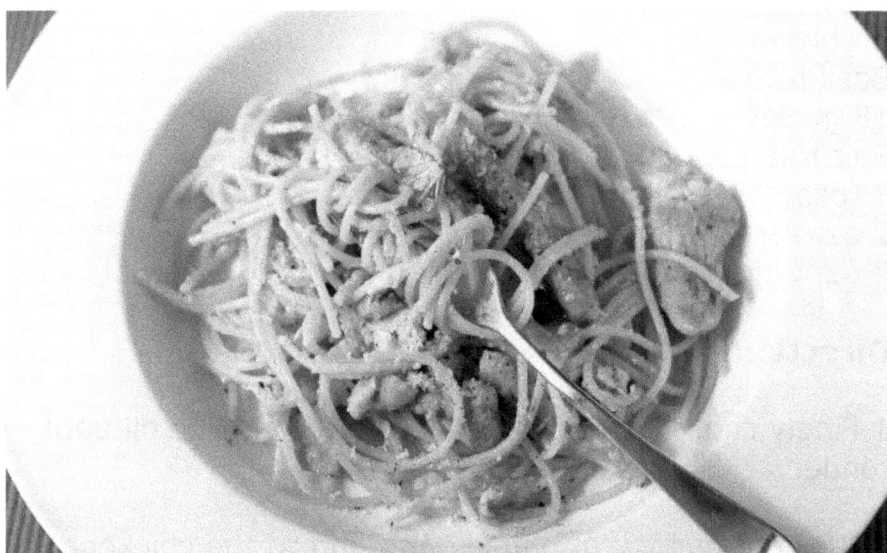

Carbonara With Fettuccine

Preparation Time: 10 minutes
Cooking Time: 25 minutes
Servings: 4

Ingredients:

17 oz. Fettuccine Pasta
8 slices Bacon
4 eggs
2 oz. Grated Parmesan Cheese
315 ml. Cream

Directions:

1.Cut the bacon into thin strips and fry in a pan over medium heat until crisp. Lay on a paper towel.

2.Put the pasta in a pot of boiling salted water and cook until cooked. Drain and return to pan.

3.While the pasta is boiling, beat the eggs with cream and parmesan until smooth. Add the bacon and mix well. Pour the sauce into a hot paste and mix well.

4.Return to a frying pan to a very small fire and simmer a little less than 1 minute until the sauce thickens slightly.

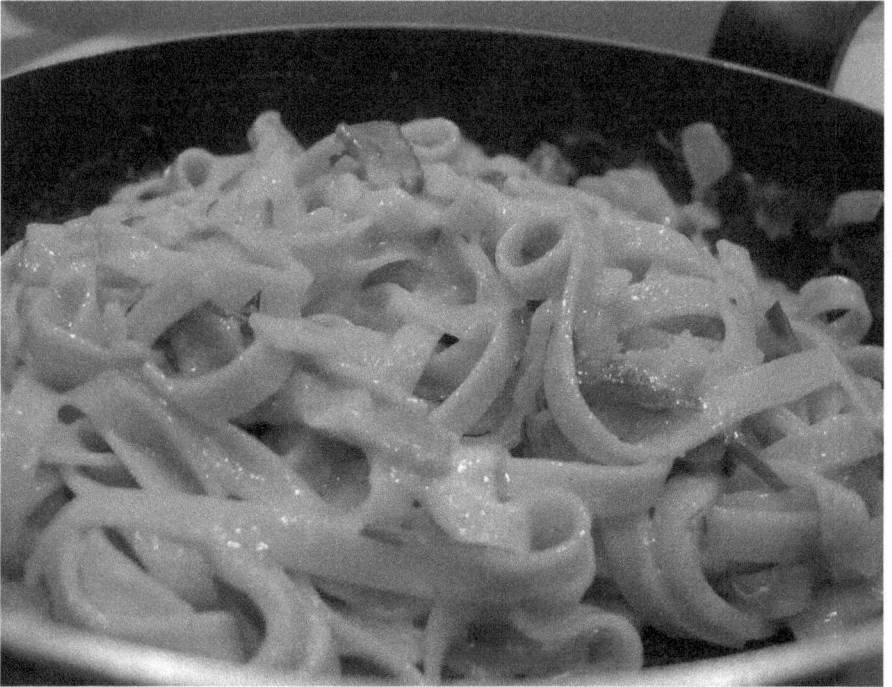

Fast Spaghetti Carbonara

Preparation Time: 5 minutes
Cooking Time: 30 minutes
Servings: 3

Ingredients:

3 oz. Spaghetti
1.5 oz. Bacon
50 ml. Cream 35%
1 pieces Chicken egg
20 ml. Dry white wine
0,8 oz. Grana padano cheese

Directions:

1.We put spaghetti in boiling water, cook for 12 minutes, put it in a sieve.

2.We separate the yolk from the Protein at the chicken egg, mix the yolks with animal cream, grana padano cheese, and pepper.

3.Cut the bacon with a large plate into large plates, fry in butter, add dry white wine and olive oil.

4.Into the fried bacon with wine and oil we introduce ready-made spaghetti, add the mass with egg and cream, mix quickly

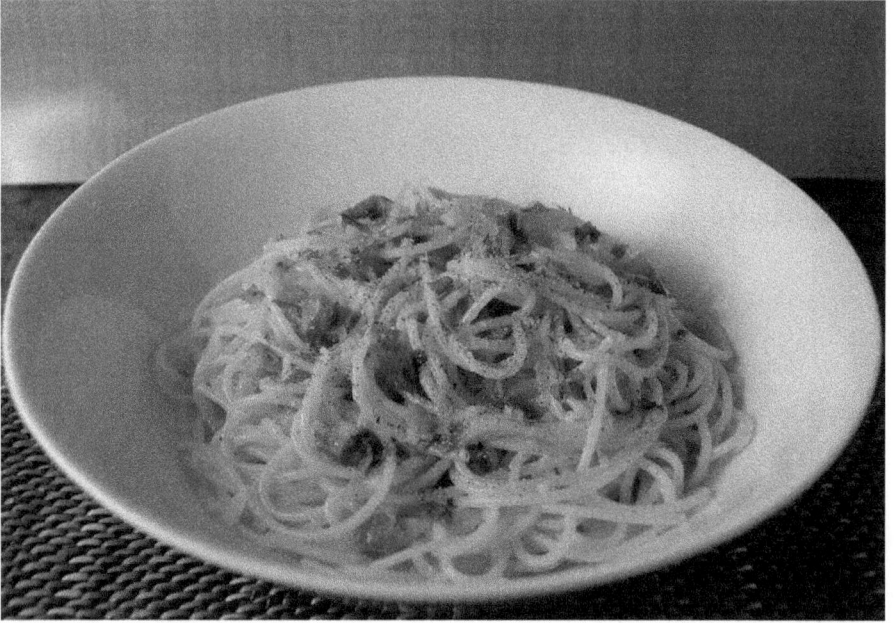

Pasta with Greens
Preparation Time: 35 Minutes
Servings: 8

Ingredients:

1 bunch Swiss chard (remove the stems)
½ cup Oil packed sun-dried tomatoes (chopped)
½ cup Green olives (chopped and pitted)
¼ cup Fresh parmesan cheese (grated)
1 package Dry fusilli pasta
2 tbsp Olive oil
½ cup Kalamata olives (chopped and pitted)
1 clove Garlic (minced)

Directions:

1.Cook pasta in lightly salted water for 10 to 12 minutes until al dente then drain.

2.Put the chard in a microwave safe bowl, fill with water until it is about ½ filled with water. Cook on high in the microwave for about 5 minutes until the chard is limp then drain.

3.Over medium heat, heat the oil in a skillet. Stir in the oil, the sun-dried tomatoes, green olives, kalamata olives and garlic.

4.Mix in the chard the cook and stir until the mixture is tender.

5.Toss with the pasta and sprinkle with parmesan cheese to serve.

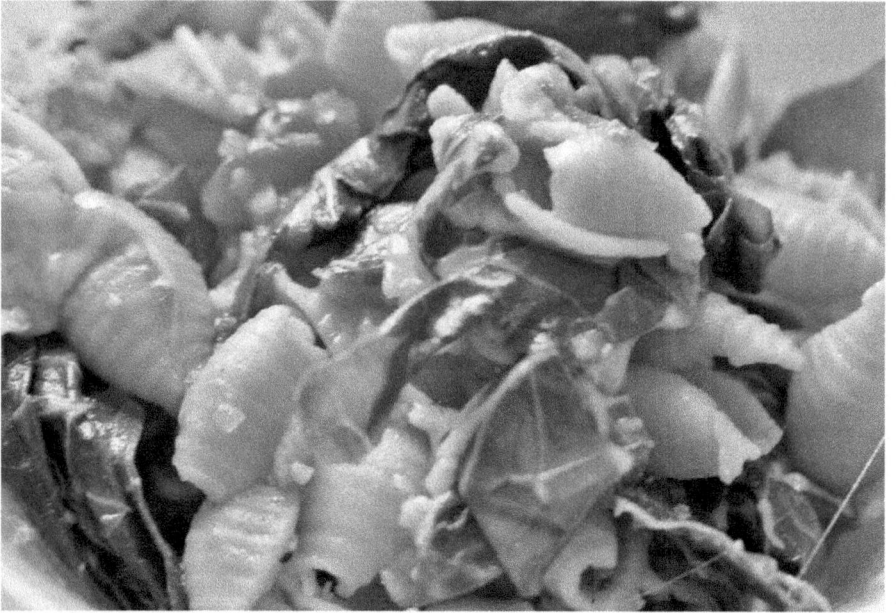

Harvest Pasta

Preparation Time: 35 minutes
Cooking Time: 4 minutes
Servings: 6

Ingredients:

1/3 cup Kalamata olives (pitted)
2 cloves Garlic (minced)
1 tbsp White sugar or more to taste
1 tsp Dried oregano
¾ cup Vegetarian burger crumbs
2 cans Diced tomatoes
1/3 cup Bottled roasted red peppers (chopped)
1 ½ tbsp Balsamic vinegar
2 tbsp Olive oil
Black pepper to taste
1 lb. Penne pasta

Directions:

1.In a large saucepan, stir the olives, garlic, sugar, oregano, tomatoes, red pepper, vinegar. Bring this to simmer for about 20 to 30 minutes over medium high-heat before reducing to medium-low and let simmer until the sauce starts to thicken.

2.In a large pot, pour lightly salted water and boil over high heat. Once the water is boiling, put in the penne pasta and leave to boil.

3.Cook the pasta uncovered for about 11 minutes and remember to stir occasionally until the pasta is al-dente. After this drain.

4.Once the tomato sauce is done, pour it into the blender no more than halfway full. Hold down the lid and carefully start the blender using a few pulses to get the sauce moving before leaving it on to puree. Afterwards, puree until the mixture is smooth, then return to the pot.

5.Stir in the burger crumbles and simmer until it is hot. Then pour the finished sauce over the penne pasta to serve.

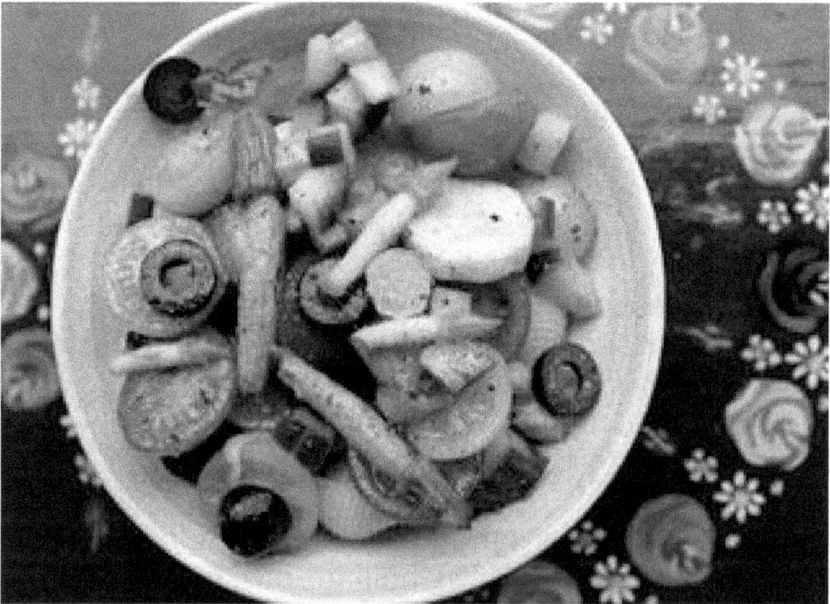

Pollo Mediterranean

Preparation Time: 25 minutes
Cooking Time: 10 minutes
Servings: 4

Ingredients:

2 tbsp. Olive oil
3 cloves Garlic (minced)
Ground black pepper
¼ cup Sun-dried tomatoes packed (chopped and drained)
½ cup Dry white wine
12 Chicken tenders (sliced into strips)
½ tsp Salt
1 tbsp Italian seasoning
2 tbsp Green olives (sliced)
2 tbsp Fresh parsley (chopped)
½ cup Sour cream
½ tsp Salt
1 cup Milk
1 ½ tsp Cornstarch
¼ cup Water

Directions:

1.In a skillet and over medium heat, heat olive oil. Place chicken and garlic in the pan. Season with pepper, Italian seasoning and ½ tsp. of salt.

2.Stir in the olives, wine, parsley, tomatoes and olives then reduce heat to a low and continue cooking until the chicken is no longer pink at the center. Remove and place chicken on a late with the sauce still in the pan.

3.Stir into the remaining sauce ½ tsp. of sauce.

4.In a small bowl, whisk cornstarch and water together. Increase heat to the medium and whisk in the cornstarch mixture. Continue stirring until the sauce has thickened. Serve the sauce with chicken.

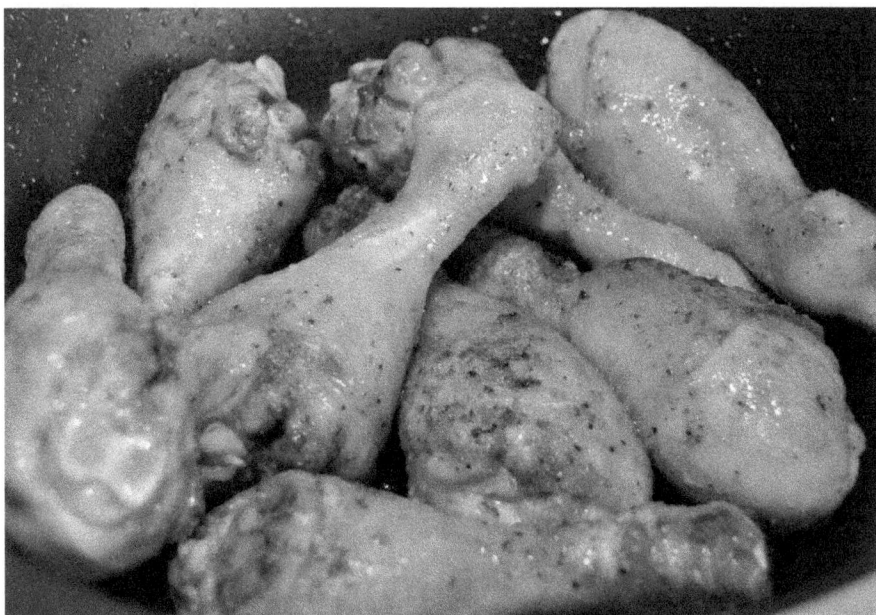

Pasta Fagioli Soup

Preparation Time: 25 minutes
Cooking Time: 35 minutes
Servings: 6

Ingredients:

3 cups Water
8 slices Crisp cooked bacon – (crumbled)
1 tbsp Dried parsley
1 tbsp Garlic (minced)
1 tsp Garlic powder
½ tsp Ground black pepper
1 ½ tsp Salt
½ tsp Dried basil
8 oz Tomato sauce can
½ lb Seashell pasta
14 oz. cans Great Northern beans (undrained)
2 cans Chicken broth
1 can Diced tomatoes
1 can Chopped spinach (drained)

Directions:

1.Combine all the other ingredients apart from pasta in a large stock pot to cook and boil. Let simmer for about 40 minutes.

2.Add pasta and cook with the pot uncovered until the pasta is tender. This should take approximately 10 minutes.

3.Serve.

Tip: You can substitute half of the canned ingredients for better nutritional outcomes.

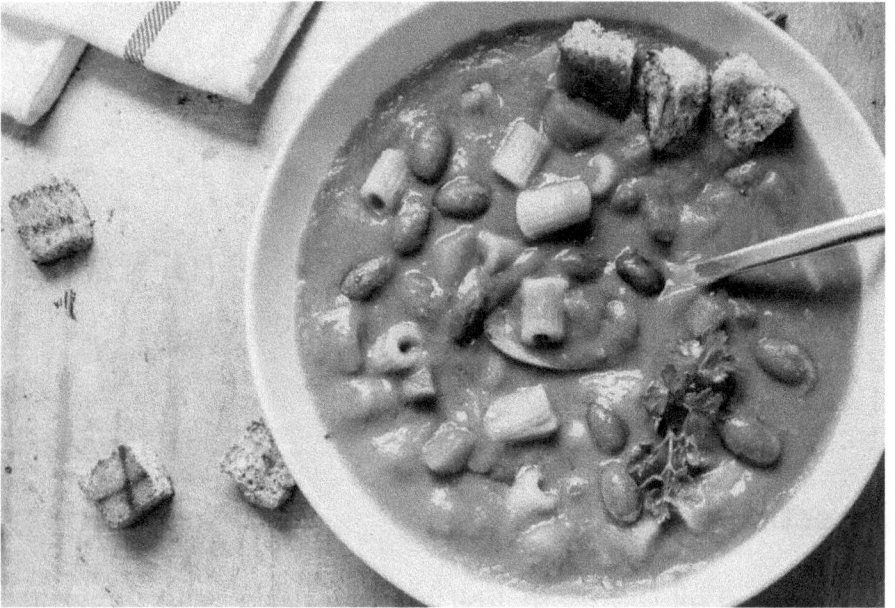

Pasta al Mediterraneo

Preparation Time: 25 minutes
Cooking Time: 15 minutes
Servings: 6

Ingredients:

1 lb. Perciatelli pasta
3 tbsp Pine nuts (lightly roasted)
2 tbsp. Fresh parsley (chopped)
1 Lemon
2 Can tuna package (drained)
12 Kalamata olives(pitted and sliced)
1 clove Garlic (crushed)
4 oz. Fresh basil (chopped)
6 tbsp Olive oil
2 oz. Feta cheese (optional)

Directions:

1.Cook pasta in a large bowl of slightly salted water until al dente. Meanwhile, mix in a large bowl, olives, garlic, basil, tuna, pine nuts, parsley and crumbled feta cheese.

2.Drain the pasta. If the plan is to serve cold, then rinse the pasta with cold water until it is no longer hot. In a large bowl, place pasta together with lemon juice and olive oil. Stir into the pasta mixture, the tuna mixture.

3.Serve hot or cold.

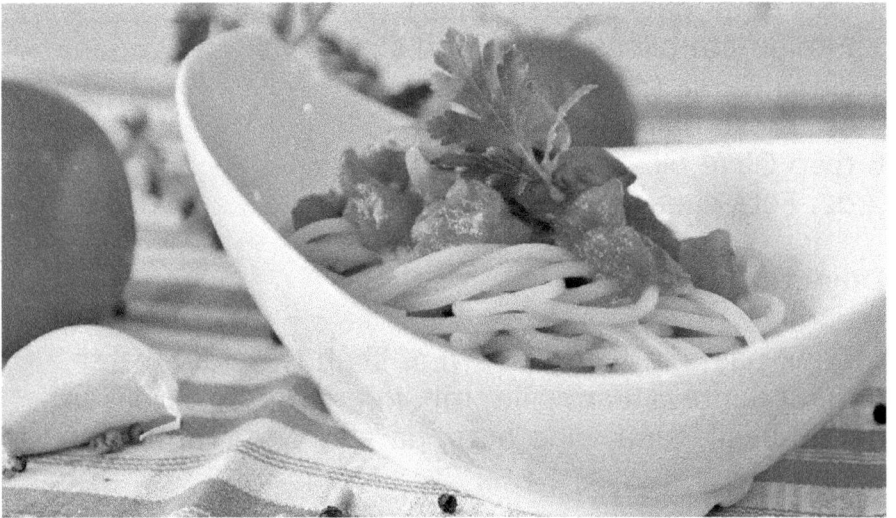

Quick Mediterranean Pasta

Preparation Time: 25 minutes
Cooking Time: 10 minutes
Servings: 6

Ingredients:

¼ cup Breadcrumbs
1 tsp Dried basil
8 oz. Spaghetti
1 tsp. Dried oregano
1 tbsp Olive oil

Directions:

1.Boil slightly salted water in a large pot, put spaghetti in it and cook until al dente. Rinse and cool with water, then drain well.

2.Mix the breadcrumbs, basil, oregano and cooked pasta in a large bowl. Pour as much olive oil as you would like over the mixture and serve.

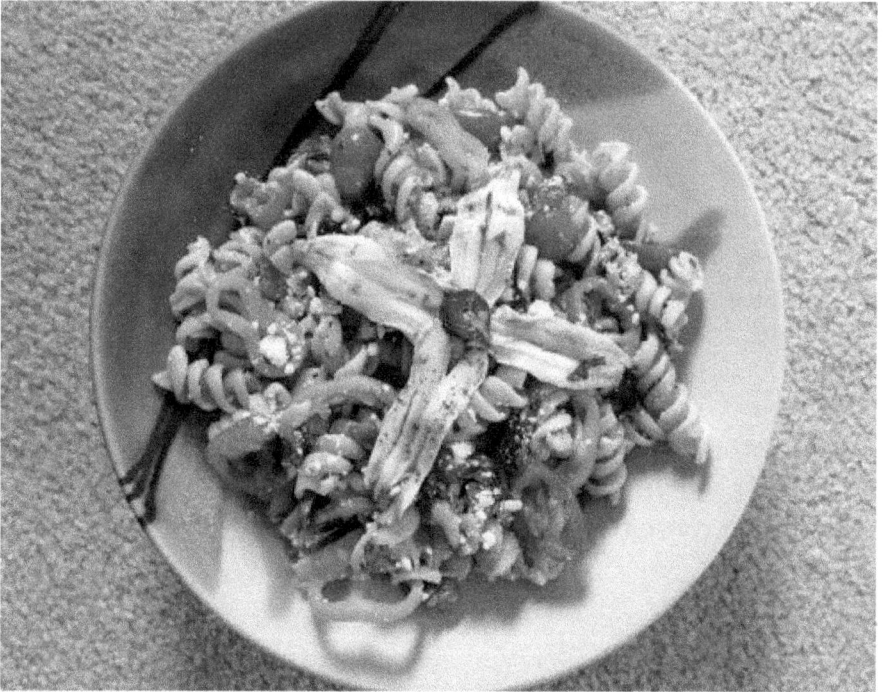

Mediterranean Fish and Pasta Stew
Preparation Time: 20 minutes
Cooking Time: 30 minutes
Servings: 4

Ingredients:

2 Onions
1 can Crushed tomatoes
½ cup Fresh parsley
2 tbsp Worcestershire sauce.
1 tsp Paprika
3 oz. Dry pasta
4 cloves Garlic (minced)
1 tbsp Olive oil
6 cups Water
½ cup Fresh cilantro (chopped)
1 tsp Ground cinnamon
1 ½ lb. Cod fillets. (cubed)
Salt to taste
1 tbsp Ground black pepper

Directions:

1.In a large pot, sauté the onions and garlic in the olive oil for 5 minutes over medium heat while stirring constantly.

2.Add tomatoes with the liquid, parsley, water and cilantro. Bring the mixture to boil and reduce heat to low and simmer for about 15 minutes.

3.Stir in the Worcestershire sauce, paprika, cinnamon and fish, the simmer over medium heat for 10 minutes.

4.Add the pasta and simmer for about 8 minutes more or until the pasta is tender.

5.Season with salt and ground pepper to taste.

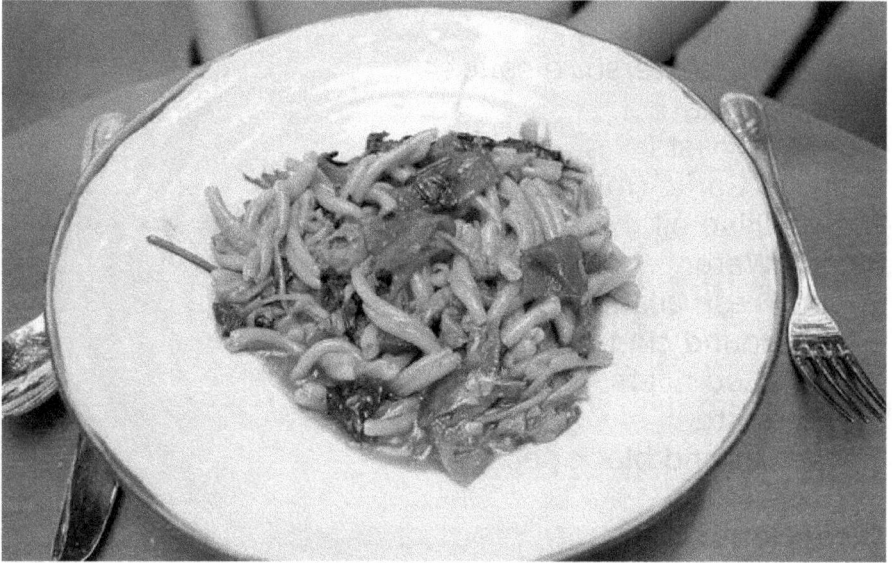

Parsley Pesto Paste

Preparation Time: 5 minutes
Cooking Time: 15 minutes
Servings: 4

Ingredients:

2 cups of parsley leaves
1/2 cup of grated parmesan cheese
2 cloves of garlic
1/2 cup lemon juice
1/4 cup olive oil
1/3 cup pine nut
Table salt to taste

Directions:

1.Put all ingredients except the parmesan cheese in a food processor then pulse until smooth.

2.Remove from the blender, add grated parmesan and gently stir.

3.Serve.

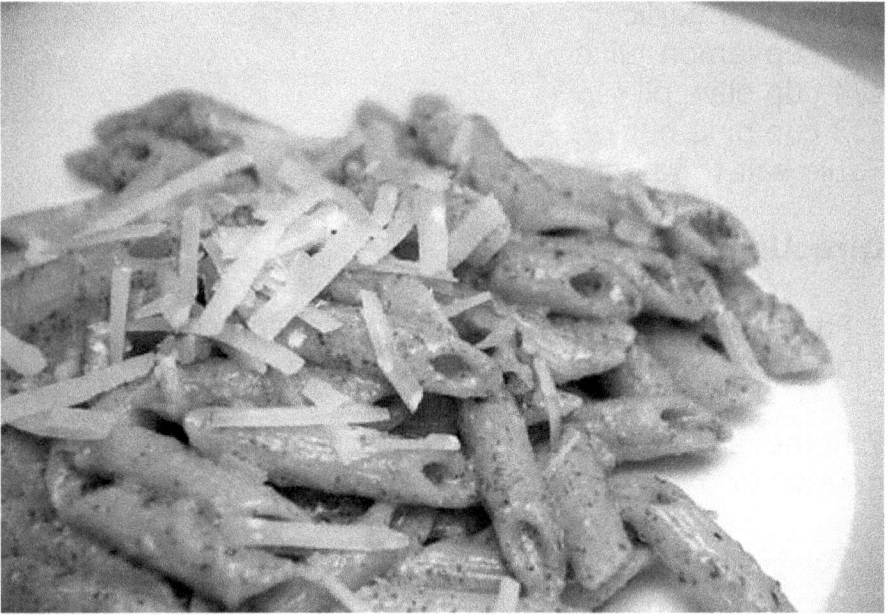

Potato in Tomato Paste

Preparation Time: 25 minutes
Cooking Time: 30 minutes
Servings: 4

Ingredients:

4 large cubed potatoes
1 Tbsp aromatic dry spices mix
1 onion, chopped
4 Tbsp Olive oil
Black pepper
1 minced garlic clove
1 cup tomato paste
1 cup of water
Chopped parsley
Salt

Directions:

1.Heat the olive oil in a pan over medium heat and sauté the onion until translucent.

2.Add the potatoes, the spice mixture and continue to sauté.

3.Add the garlic, tomato paste, diced tomato, water, salt and pepper, and stir.

4.Cover the pot and cook for half an hour over low heat.

5.Serve with fresh coriander.

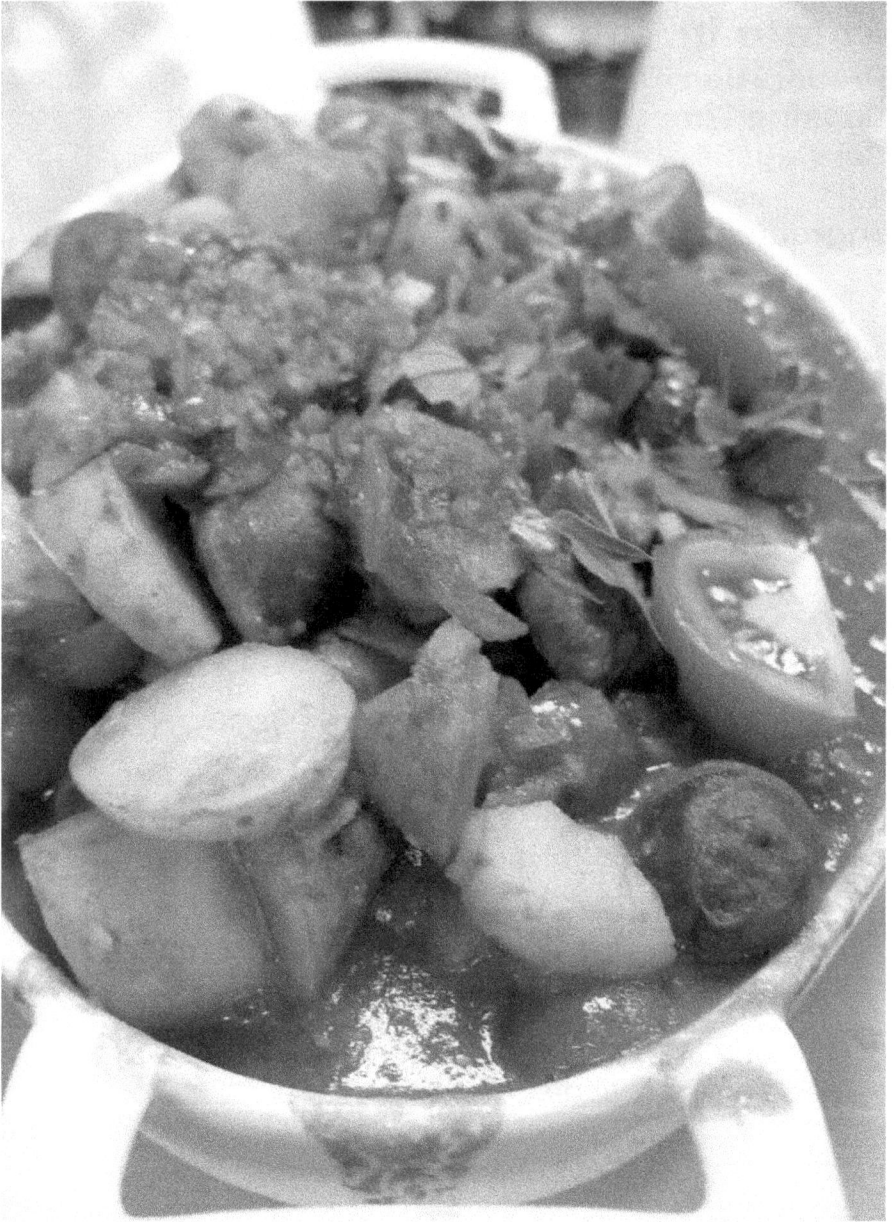

Hummus

Preparation Time: 15 minutes
Cooking Time: 10 minutes
Servings: 4

Ingredients:

1/2 cup tahini
1 tsp salt
2 cloves garlic halved
1 tbsp olive oil
2 cup canned garbanzo beans, drained
1/2 cup lemon juice
1 tbsp paprika
1 tsp parsley

Directions:

1.Pulse the garlic, lemon juice, garbanzos, salt, and tahini in a food processor until smooth.

2.Add this to a bowl with olive oil, paprika, and parsley.

3.Enjoy.

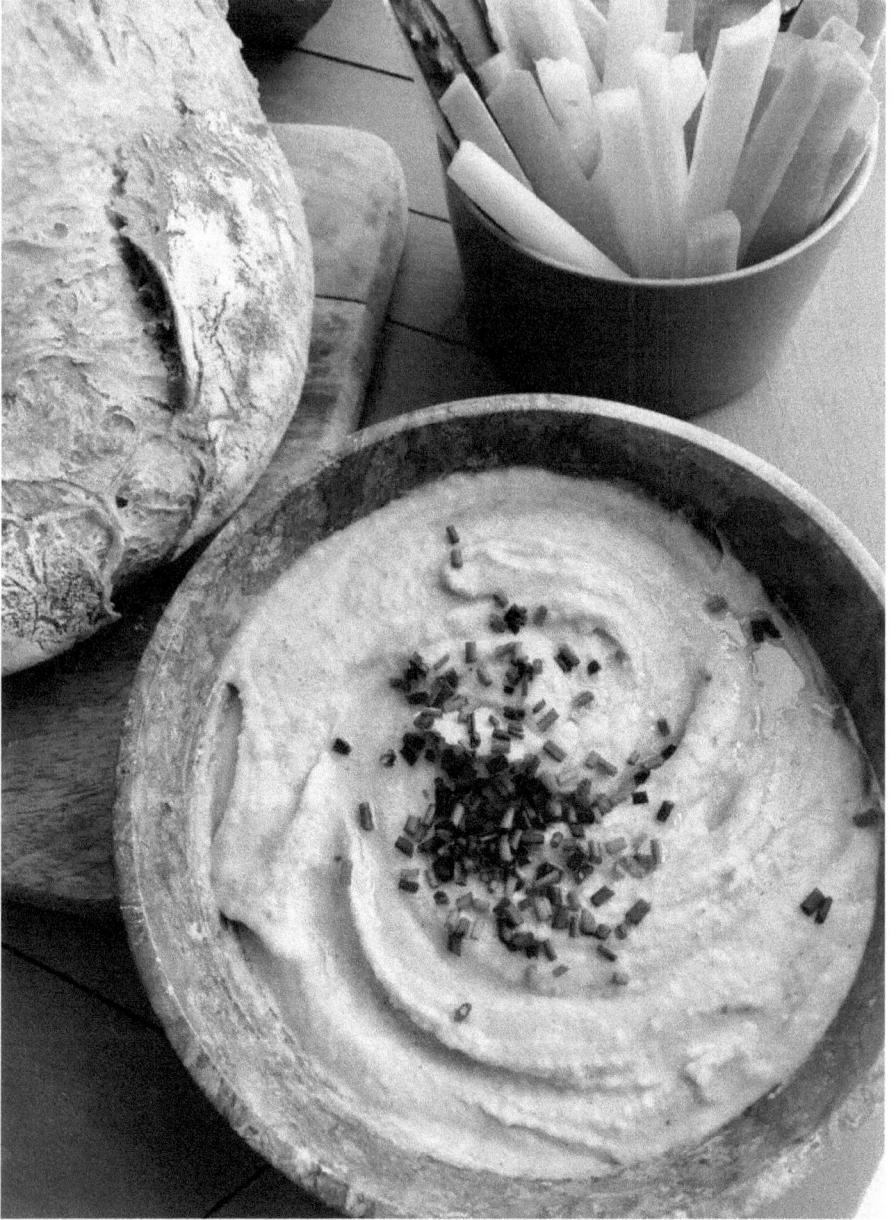